NEUROLOGY - LABORATORY AND CLINICAL RESEARCH DEVELOPMENTS

HYPERHIDROSIS

CAUSES, TREATMENT OPTIONS AND OUTCOMES

NEUROLOGY - LABORATORY AND CLINICAL RESEARCH DEVELOPMENTS

Additional books in this series can be found on Nova's website under the Series tab.

Additional e-books in this series can be found on Nova's website under the e-book tab.

NEUROLOGY - LABORATORY AND CLINICAL RESEARCH DEVELOPMENTS

HYPERHIDROSIS

CAUSES, TREATMENT OPTIONS AND OUTCOMES

JANINE R. HUDDLE
EDITOR

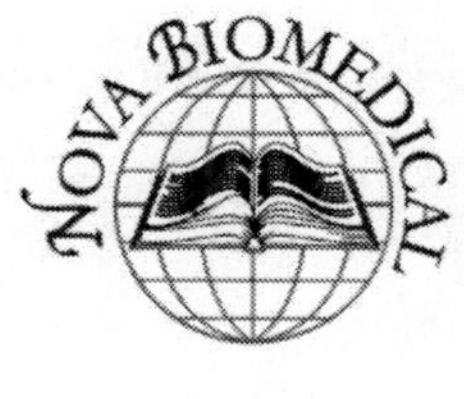

New York

For permission to use material from this book please contact us:
Telephone 631-231-7269; Fax 631-231-8175
Web Site: http://www.novapublishers.com

Library of Congress Cataloging-in-Publication Data

ISBN: 978-1-63321-516-0

Library of Congress Control Number: 2014944806

Published by Nova Science Publishers, Inc. † New York

Contents

Preface

An estimated 7.8 million Americans suffer from hyperhidrosis with up to 1.3 million reporting severe disease. Affected patients can experience limitations in occupational and social circumstances. As a result, patients with hyperhidrosis often experience decreased physical and emotional wellbeing, difficulty in personal relationships, and can suffer from social stigmatization. This book discusses several different causes of hyperhidrosis, as well as treatment options and outcomes.

Chapter I – Hyperhidrosis is defined as excessive sweat production beyond requirements for temperature regulation. It can be idiopathic, secondary to other systemic conditions such as endocrine or autonomic dysfunction, as well as a side effect to medication. Botulinum toxin type A is a safe and effective treatment option for patients suffering from focal hyperhidrosis, producing longer-lasting symptom relief than topical therapies and obviating the need for invasive surgical procedures. The toxin can be administered in a minimally invasive manner via injection. Effects of treatment are fairly durable, lasting from six to nine months on average with high patient satisfaction. Greatest success has been reported for the use of botulinum toxin to treat hyperhidrosis in the axillary region; however palmar, plantar, and even craniofacial hyperhidrosis can also benefit from treatment. Considerable debate exists in the field regarding the best timing and frequency of treatment with botulinum toxin for hyperhidrosis, and repeated injections have not been associated with attenuation of effectiveness. In this chapter, author hope to detail the optimal technique for administering botulinum toxin for hyperhidrosis and discuss the challenges and limitations of its use. Ultimately, botulinum toxin injection can be a safe and effective non-surgical option for long-term management of hyperhidrosis.

Chapter II – The physiopathology of primary hyperhidrosis is not completely understood: eccrine sweat glands are normal in number, size, and function in hyperhidrotic patients. Nevertheless, such patients show abnormal sympathetic skin response, suggesting that the cause of hyperhidrosis may be related to a sympathetic nervous system (which innervates eccrine sweat glands) dysfunction. Despite the resection of thoracic sympathetic chain ganglia be a treatment for primary hyperhidrosis, the function of sympathetic ganglia in normal individuals and in hyperhidrotic patients remained unknown until a short time ago. The author's studies showed abnormalities in size, ganglion cells count, collagen fibers (using picrosirius staining)/elastic fibers (using Weigert's resorcin-fuchsin method) ratio, apoptosis (using caspase-3 assay), expression of acetylcholine, and expression of a specific subunit of nicotinic acetylcholine receptor in sympathetic ganglia of hyperhidrotic patients. Such results confirm the premise that sympathetic ganglia play an important role in the pathophysiology of primary hyperhidrosis and may indicate new treatment modalities for this condition.

Chapter III – Hyperhidrosis can be a debilitating condition that affects patient's quality of life. Despite numerous non-surgical alternatives in the treatment algorithm, division of thoracic sympathetic nerves by surgery remains the most definitive treatment option and provides long-lasting results. The history of surgical sympathectomy goes back several decades, however, the access trauma of thoracotomy was a significant drawback and the main resistance to the popularization of the procedure. The invention of thoracoscopes and subsequently the development of minimal invasive thoracoscopic sympathectomy saw the increasing acceptance of the technique by patients for treatment of hyperhidrosis. The last decade has seen the surgery evolving from 3-ports to single port access, and use of 10mm thoracoscopes and instruments to the needlescopic 3mm wide instruments, which improve aesthetics and patient satisfaction with promising therapeutic results. The development of embryonic natural orifice transluminal endoscopic surgery (E-NOTES) thoracic sympathectomy holds promise in further reducing access trauma. Despite the emergence of new minimally invasive techniques, many questions concerning surgical sympathectomy remain unanswered. Issues including the level at which sympathetic interruption should occur, and how the interruption should be achieved (sympathectomy, sympathicotomy or clipping) are explored in this chapter. Furthermore, author are only just beginning to understand the undesirable effects of thoracic sympathectomy and potential surgical remedies available. The chapter will review the available literature, and share the authors' experiences on these important issues relating to thoracoscopic sympathectomy.

Chapter IV – Hyperhidrosis is a common condition which is troublesome for patients and carries a significant psychosocial burden. Hyperhidrosis can be either generalised of focal. Treatment may require oral anticholinergic agents. Focal hyperhidrosis is usually primary and responds to topical measures. Specialist referral for botulinum toxin A, iontophoresis or sympathectomy should be considered for severe cases. This article details an approach to the assessment and managment of hyperhidrosis and outlines the current treatment options that are available.

Chapter V – Primary focal hyperhidrosis is a common disorder with significant impact on occupational, physical, emotional and social life. A systematic review of current literature for primary focal hyperhidrosis was performed with focus on guidelines, epidemiology and quality of life instruments. The relation between treatment option, quality of life outcome, measured as Hyperhidrosis Disease Severity Scale (HDSS) or Dermatology Life Quality Index (DLQI), and rare treatment costs have been investigated. There are numerous instruments available to measure the quality of life (QOL) of the hyperhidrosis patient. In practice, however, only a few (HDSS, DLQI) are used. Additionally, treatment with Botulinum Toxin A seems to be the cheapest for primary focal hyperhidrosis. No relationship of cost-effectiveness and decision-making process for hyperhidrosis treatment choice could be found. For future decision-making processes the dermatologist remains to evaluate not only the severity of hyperhidrosis to achieve the best therapeutic outcome, but also to measure quality of life in order to justify patient´s expenses for treatment performance.

Chapter VI – Sweating helps to regulate body temperature by cooling via the evaporation of sweat produced by sweat glands. Hyperhidrosis is a condition characterized by constant and increased production of sweat by sweat glands, and may be local (primary) or generalized (secondary). Primary hyperhidrosis is a constant and excessive sweating disorder, of unknown cause, that occurs mainly in the axilla, palms, soles of feet and craniofacial region, and more than one area may be involved. The secondary form is caused by a latent condition, such as an infection, endocrine or metabolic disorder, neoplasic disease, neurological condition, psychiatric disorder, spinal cord injury and respiratory or cardiovascular problems. Hyperhidrosis is a clinical manifestation that significantly interferes in an individual's life, causing emotional and social problems, a lower quality of life, physical discomfort and increased risk of skin infections. In general treatment is symptomatic, and varies according to the intensity of the disease. In less severe cases it is customary to use creams and antiperspirant deodorants based on aluminium chloride. In intermediate cases the treatment of choice is oxybutynin. Severe cases require invasive modes of therapy, and are more likely in the adult population.

The most widely used form of treatment is thoracic sympathectomy, but most patients experience recurrence of the manifestation in another region of the body (compensatory hyperhidrosis or reflex) after surgery, in the absence of full resolution. The application of botulinum toxin is an alternative approach, although sweating is only temporarily reduced. Acupuncture is a form of treatment that has been used with success, because this condition, according to Traditional Chinese Medicine, is caused by a disorder in the metabolism of water, which is responsible for sweat. As acupuncture is based on treating the cause and not just the effect of pathologies, patients who undergo this treatment report a very satisfactory and more efficient outcome compared to those previously cited.

Chapter VII – Primary palmar hyperhidrosis (PPHH) is a highly disturbing pathology affecting 0.15-0.25% of the young population, ensuing severe functional and social handicaps. For decades, the second thoracic ganglion (T2) was considered to be responsible for palmar perspiration and its resection was accepted as the golden standard for the surgical treatment of PPHH. However, sympathetic ablation bears several sequels, compensatory hyperhidrosis (CHH) being the gravest and most commonly observed. It consists in increased perspiration of a part of the body unaffected by the sympathetic ablation, and may attain devastating proportions. The mechanism of CCH is complex, enigmatic and obscure. To reduce its magnitude, two major approached were suggested: (a) modification of the surgical procedure by clipping or transecting the sympathetic chain instead of resecting the ganglion, and/or lowering the level of the procedure from T2 to T3-T4; and (b) reversal procedures: unclipping or reconstructing the continuity of the sympathetic chain by nerve grafting. The actual consensus is that appropriate sympathetic ablation is the only treatment which may cure PPHH. All methods of performing the procedure are still debated as are the proposed approaches to reduce CHH.

The methods by which results are evaluated are also controversial. QoL is examined by questionnaires, several types of which have been proposed. Comparing QoL before and after surgical sympathetic ablation is usually the method of evaluating results in use.

However, this is a subjective method and no comparison of results of different studies is possible. Furthermore, to learn the pathophysiological aspects of a surgical procedure, metrical assessment of results is required. The aim of the present report is to review the literature and present the State of the Art concerning the surgical treatment of PPHH.

In: Hyperhidrosis
Editor: Janine R. Huddle

ISBN: 978-1-63321-516-0

Chapter I

Botulinum Toxin for the Treatment of Primary Focal Hyperhidrosis: Pretreatment Considerations, Technique and Expected Outcomes

Naikhoba C. O. Munabi*[1]*, B.A.,
Jeffrey A. Ascherman*[1]*, M.D.,
and Melissa A. Doft*[2]*, M.D.,
[1]Division of Plastic Surgery, Columbia University Medical Center, New York-Presbyterian Hospital, New York, NY, US
[2]Division of Plastic Surgery, Weill Cornell Medical Center, New York-Presbyterian Hospital, New York, NY, US

Abstract

Hyperhidrosis is defined as excessive sweat production beyond requirements for temperature regulation. It can be idiopathic, secondary to other systemic conditions such as endocrine or autonomic dysfunction, as well as a side effect to medication. Botulinum toxin type A is a safe and effective treatment option for patients suffering from focal hyperhidrosis, producing longer-lasting symptom relief than topical therapies and obviating the need for invasive surgical procedures. The toxin can be administered in a minimally invasive manner via injection. Effects of treatment are fairly durable, lasting from six to nine months on average with high patient satisfaction. Greatest success has been reported for the use of botulinum toxin to treat hyperhidrosis in the axillary region; however palmar, plantar, and even craniofacial hyperhidrosis can also benefit from treatment. Considerable debate exists in the field regarding the best timing and frequency of treatment with botulinum toxin for hyperhidrosis, and repeated injections have not been associated with attenuation of effectiveness. In this chapter, we hope to detail the optimal technique for administering botulinum toxin for hyperhidrosis and discuss the challenges and limitations of its use. Ultimately, botulinum toxin injection can be a safe and effective non-surgical option for long-term management of hyperhidrosis.

Introduction

Hyperhidrosis is a condition resulting in excessive sweating beyond normal requirements for body temperature regulation. An estimated 7.8 million Americans suffer from hyperhidrosis with up to 1.3 million reporting severe disease. [1] Affected patients can experience limitations in occupational and social circumstances. As a result, patients with hyperhidrosis often experience decreased physical and emotional wellbeing, difficulty in personal relationships, and can suffer from social stigmatization. [2-6]

Primary hyperhidrosis can be treated both surgically and non-surgically. Surgical treatment options include endoscopic transthoracic sympathectomy (ETC), arthroscopic shaving of sweat glands, and excision of the glands. Though they can be temporarily effective, these treatments are invasive and can be associated with serious complications and high recurrence rates. [7-11] Additionally, operative costs, anesthesia, and surgical recovery time make a surgical approach to treatment less ideal. [7-11] First-line non-surgical treatment options include topical antiperspirants such as aluminum chloride. Effects, however, are short acting requiring frequent reapplication, can be intolerable due to irritant dermatitis, and may be ineffective in reducing sweat production.. [12,13]

Botulinum toxin type A has recently emerged as an effective treatment for focal hyperhidrosis, and has been shown to be safer and less invasive than surgery, while also providing more tolerable and longer-lasting relief of symptoms than current topical treatment options. [14] Botulinum toxin type A, commonly known under the trade name Botox, is one of four FDA approved botulinum toxins, but was the first to be proposed for treatment of focal hyperhidrosis after it was observed to inhibit sweat production in healthy patients. [15, 16] The toxin functions by temporarily inhibiting the release of acetylcholine, thereby preventing the hyperstimulation of eccrine sweat glands that leads to excessive sweating. [17] Several randomized studies have supported that botulinum toxin type A is a safe, effective, and long-lasting treatment option for patients with primary hyperhidrosis. [2, 3, 12, 17-23] In fact, when patients who have been unresponsive to topical antiperspirants are injected with botulinum toxin, research has shown they experience a 75% reduction in sweating [21], improved emotional and physical wellbeing [19], and decreased activity limitations [23] without experiencing any serious adverse events. In our experience, we have observed a reduction in reported symptoms within two weeks of treatment and persisting for an average period of six to nine months, as well as high patient satisfaction rates. [24] Recent studies have suggested that other botulinum toxins may also be safe and effective in the treatment of focal hyperhidrosis. [25-27] In this chapter, however, we will focus predominantly on botulinum toxin type A with the primary goal to provide guidance on the appropriate preoperative evaluation, injection technique, and the anticipated outcomes after treatment.

Diagnosis

Primary hyperhidrosis is defined as idiopathic and excessive sweating lasting six months or more with at least two of the following features: frequency greater than once a week, impairment of daily activity, symmetric sweating bilaterally, onset prior to age 25, positive family history, and cessation of focal symptoms while sleeping. [6, 14] Focal disease is typically localized to the axillae, palms, and soles without widespread autonomic dysfunction. Heat, spicy foods, and emotional triggers can exacerbate symptoms, though the condition is not considered a psychiatric disorder. The exact etiology of the condition is unclear; however, hyperhidrosis is believed to result from a non-thermoregulatory sympathetic hyperstimulation of eccrine sweat glands with a possible autosome dominant hereditary pattern. [28, 29]

Primary hyperhidrosis is diagnosed clinically based on the severity of daily impairment from the sweating disorder. Patient history is critical to determining the degree of severity. Typically, patients report onset of excessive sweating symptoms beginning in childhood or adolescence. Despite the fact that the majority of patients suffer from idiopathic disease, possible diagnoses resulting in secondary hyperhidrosis symptoms should be considered in all patients, such as underlying malignancy, infection, endocrine and neurological disorders, or medication side effects. [30] Even more rarely, patients may suffer from focal hyperhidrosis related to a specific syndrome, such as Ross syndrome, Frey syndrome, or localized unilateral hyperhidrosis.

Pretreatment Evaluation

Both objective and subjective measures have been developed to assist in determining the severity of excessive sweat production and the degree of patient impairment. Objective measurements for focal sweating disorders include the Minor's starch iodine test and gravimetry. In the Minor's test, a 3.5% iodine in alcohol solution is applied to clean, shaved, and dried skin of the affected area. Standard starch flour is then sprinkled on top of the iodine solution. As sweat contacts the iodine-starch mixture, a color change occurs producing a dark violet pigment. This color change assists in diagraming the distribution of active eccrine glands in the affected area, which can further guide the appropriate area to treat. [14, 31]

Gravimetry is the gold standard and most commonly used objective measurement for assessing focal hyperhidrosis. Filter paper is weighed prior to and after exposure to the affected area of skin for a defined period of time (60 seconds or 5 minutes). The weight difference quantifies the amount of sweat produced over a period of time. This measurement can be further normalized by the area of sweat production. In healthy volunteers, gravimetry measurements were found to be 25, 66, and 153 mg/min/m^2 for the facial, axillary and palmar regions respectively. [32] For axillary hyperhidrosis, diagnosis is typically associated with a gravimetry measurement of >50 mg/min. [2]

Though objective measurements are helpful for diagnosis and research purposes, the decision to pursue treatment and evaluation of treatment effectiveness is largely based on patient reported quality-of-life and perceived impairment. For that reason, subjective measurements tend to be more valuable and easier to determine in the office setting. Two questionnaires are commonly used for subjectively assessing the quality-of-life impairment from hyperhidrosis and tracking responsiveness to treatment. The Dermatology Life Quality Index (DLQI) is a validated measure consisting of 10 questions each scored from 0-3 with a maximum overall score of 30 and minimum score of 0. Higher scores suggest greater impact of symptoms from a skin disease on quality-of-life. [33, 34] The Hyperhidrosis Disease Severity Scale (HDSS) is, as suggested in its name, specific to the effects of hyperhidrosis on a patient's life. The scale assesses tolerability of symptoms and the degree to which they interfere with daily life. A higher HDSS score, which ranges from 1 to 4, indicates a greater interference of symptoms. [35] The HDSS was designed for axillary hyperhidrosis; however, the gradation scale can be extrapolated to other focal symptoms. [35] In our experience, we have preferred to use the HDSS as opposed to the DLQI for assessing disease severity of hyperhidrosis.

Patients frequently are plagued by the psychosocial sequelae of hyperhidrosis, leading to anxiety, decreased socialization, and difficulty in personal and occupational situations. [2-6] As a result, patients either self-refer or are referred by their primary care physicians to the plastic surgeon's office. In our practice, we have used botulinum toxin to treat patients who are older than age 14 and suffer from persistent primary hyperhidrosis. Prior to injection, however, patients must demonstrate failure of response or intolerance to nonsurgical treatment options such as topical antiperspirants for all focal regions, or tap water iontophoresis for the palmar and plantar regions. Tap water iontophoresis temporarily disrupts ion channels by passing a direct current through an electrolyte solution in contact with moisturized pedals on the skin, and is an accepted nonsurgical option for treating palmoplantar hyperhidrosis. [36] Two weeks of treatment is typically sufficient to test the efficacy of topical agents. Botulinum toxin injection is offered as a treatment for patients who are refractory or intolerant to nonsurgical treatment options, and those who score a three or four on the HDSS scale. Such an HDSS score indicates that the patient's symptoms are minimally tolerable and are interfering with daily activities. This treatment strategy is in line with the recommended treatment approach by the Canadian Hyperhidrosis Advisory Committee, which advises topical treatment for HDSS scores of 2 and below, and recommends either topical or botulinum toxin as first line therapy for HDSS scores of 3 and 4. [37] All patients undergo standard pretreatment counseling with discussion of the risks, benefits, and alternative treatment options.

Contraindications

Botulinum toxin injections are not offered to patients who suffer from hyperhidrosis secondary to an underling medical condition. Treatment should be considered with caution in patients who have undergone previous surgical debulking of sweat glands, or who have severe comorbidities. [25] Patients with a concurrent infection at the injection site or systemic infection are requested to return to the office after resolution of the infection. Treatment should be avoided in patients with an existing medical condition that may interfere with neuromuscular function, such as myasthenia gravis, Lambert-Eaton syndrome, or amyotrophic lateral sclerosis. Female patients who are pregnant or breastfeeding are also excluded from treatment.

Technique

Botox Solution

Botulinum toxin (BTX) is a neurotoxin derived from the anaerobic bacterium, *Clostridium botulinum*, that functions by temporarily binding to acetylcholine receptors on the presynaptic membrane and subsequently blocking the release of acetylcholine from skeletal and autonomic cholinergic nerve terminals. Therefore, in hyperhidrosis botulinum toxin results in chemodenervation of the eccrine glands leading to attenuation of symptoms.

Each serotype of botulinum toxin is antigenically distinct; however, all have similar molecular weights with a common subunit. [38] Of the seven known serotypes of botulinum toxin (A, B, C, D, E, F, and G), only four serotypes (A, B, E, and F) have known poisonous effects on humans. Multiple international studies of serotype A (BTX-A) in the formulation of Botox (Allergan, Inc., Irvine, California) or Dysport (Ipsen, Brisbane, California) have demonstrated safety and efficacy for numerous indications. [39] Both products are based off of the BTX-A serotype but have different dosing protocols, and thus cannot be used interchangeably at the same dose. Currently onaboulinumtoxinA (BoNT-ONA; Botox) is the only US Food and Drug Administration (FDA)-approved BTX-A formulation of the treatment of hyperhidrosis. A third formulation of BTX-A, Xeromin (incobotulinumtoxinA, Merz, Greenborough, North Carolina), has recently been FDA-approved for cosmetic use and has been suggested as another potential treatment for hyperhidrosis; however, further studies are needed to confirm dosing and efficacy. [40] BTX-B, available as Neurobloc (Elan Pharmaceuticals, Dublin, Ireland) and Myobloc (Solstice Neurosciences, LLC., San Francisco, CA) have been shown to also be effective in the treatment of axillary and palmar hyperhidrosis, especially for patients who do not respond to BTX-A therapy. [41-44] In a case study of 10 patients who received BTX-A treatment in one axilla and BTX-B treatment in the other, BTX-B was significantly more effective in reducing sweat production and area compared to BTX-A. Effects of treatment were also seen earlier with BTX-B and patients reported significantly greater satisfaction. [44] Despite reports of greater effectiveness, BTX-B is associated with a different and more extensive side effect profile than BTX-A, with more regional pain and irritation at the injection site, as well as increased reports of systemic anticholinergic adverse effects. [44, 45] For these reasons, in our practice we use BTX-A.

We prepare and administer BoNT-ONA diluted in a sterile saline solution at a concentration of 1 mL of saline for every 25 U of BoNT-ONA (Table 1). Some authors add lidocaine to the solution to reduce the pain associated with injections. [46] Standard doses of BoNT-ONA include 50 U for each axilla, 100 U for each palm, and 150 U for each sole. In our practice, we have injected up to 200 U in one treatment session. FDA recommendations state that treatment should not exceed a 360 U cumulative dose in a three-month period.

Table 1. Botulinum Toxin Type A Reconstitution

Parameter	Recommendation
Diluent	0.9% saline solution
Concentration	25 U botulinum toxin to 1 mL 0.9% saline solution
Axillary dilution	50 U botulinum toxin in 2 mL saline per axilla (3 mL for larger axillae); 40 injections per milliliter of injection solution
Palmar dilution	100 U botulinum toxin in 3-4 mL saline per palm
Plantar dilution	150-250 U botulinum toxin in 6-8 mL saline per sole

Axillary Treatment

Prior to beginning treatment, the affected hyperhidrotic area must be identified. Some authors administer the Minor's starch iodine test to delineate the location of sweat glands in the axilla. The appropriate area for treatment, however, can also be defined according to the hear-bearing area in the axilla, and delineated with a marking pen prior to administration of a betadine prep (Figure 1).

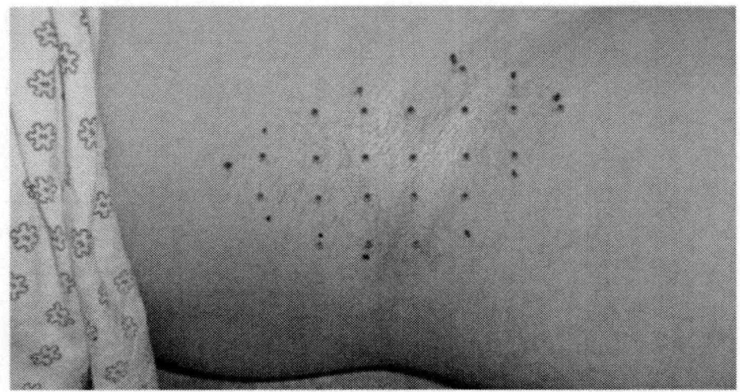

Figure 1. The hair-bearing area is delineated with a marking pen (purple dots at periphery). These markings can be imagined as a grid of injection sites (green dots).

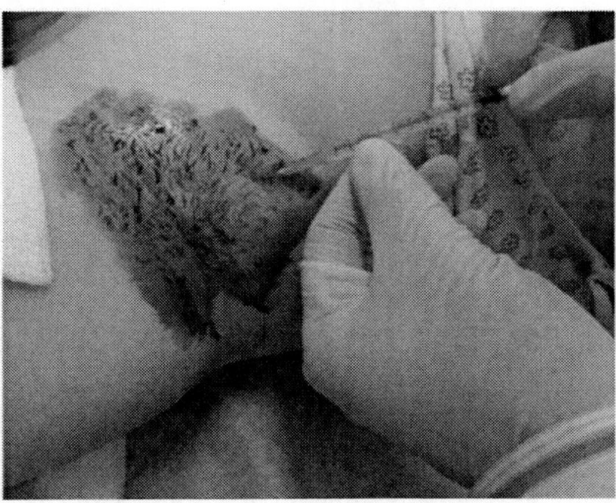

Figure 2. A 26- or 30-guage needle on a TB syringe is used for injections. Injections are plasced subdermally in each axilla, with injection sites approximately 8 mm apart. During injection, the needle is inserted at a 45-degree angle approximately 2 mm into the dermis, bevel side up. Once inserted, the syringe is slowly depressed to deposit approximately 0.05 mL of the botulinum toxin solution subdermally before it is withdrawn.

Botulinum toxin can be injected into the axillary area using a 26- or 30-gauge needle on a TB syringe. In most patients, 40 evenly distributed injections (20 injections per milliliter of injection solution, or 0.05 mL of solution per injection) are placed subdermally in each axilla approximately 8 mm apart. Injection technique involves inserting the needle at a 45-degree angle, approximately 2 mm into the dermis (Figure 2). After insertion, the syringe is slowly depressed to deposit the appropriate amount of solution subdermally, after which it is withdrawn. Each injection should be performed in one smooth motion to minimize trauma to the area.

50 U of reconstituted BoNT-ONA is used in total for each axilla, as the dose was found to be the minimal dose necessary to cause anhidrosis in healthy volunteers. [15] Although for most patients 50 U can be adequately diluted into 2 mL of normal saline, occasionally a dilution volume of 3 mL is used for patients with larger axillae.

Palmar and Plantar Treatment

Both palmar and planter hyperhidrosis involve a thick epidermis, making topical agents even less effective. Both regions have abundant nerve endings, making them particularly sensitive, so the pain associated with BoNT-ONA injections can be a deterrent for many patients to undergo the procedure in these areas, considering the number of injections needed to achieve the desired effect. In an attempt to reduce the discomfort associated with injections several anesthetic methods have been reported, including oral and intravenous sedation, topical lidocaine cream, nerve blocks, Bier block, Dermojet (AKRA, Pau, France), and cryoanesthesia (ice block). [47] Radial and ulnar nerve blocks, when properly administered, are highly effective in minimizing pain and are common anesthetic choices for use prior to injection. However, not all physicians can reliably perform the procedure and there is an added risk that temporary or permanent nerve damage can occur. Additionally, many patients object to having a temporarily disabled hand. Dermojet is a device that non-invasively administers anesthesia by using air pressure to inject 2% lidocaine. This anesthetic approach, however, requires numerous injections since the physician must stop after treatment of four or five sites to ensure that botulinum toxin is administered only in the limited area penetrated with the Dermojet. [48]

For minimizing pain while treating palmoplantar hyperhidrosis, we prefer to use cryoanalgesia due to its low risk, effectiveness, minimal cost, and convenience. Ice packs are placed on the treatment area 15 minutes prior to injection for cooling. For patients who are particularly sensitive or concerned about the pain associated with the injection, a topical 2.5% lidocaine cream can also be applied 30 to 60 minutes prior to the procedure. Some physicians also use vibration, administered with a handheld massager or similar device, in conjunction with ice packs to reduce pain. It is theorized that stimulation of vibration receptors leads to inhibition of the neurons that transmit the pain signal. [49]

Similar to the treatment approach detailed for the axilla, a Minor's iodine test is typically avoided for the palmar and plantar regions for several reasons, including that patients dislike the iodine-related staining of their hands. The area of injection is defined as a grid on the palm and sole. For the palm, 100 U of BoNT-ONA diluted in 3 to 4 ml of normal saline is injected using a 26- or 30- gauge needle and a TB syringe. Injections are subdermal into each 1-cm square area of the palm and three sites on each digit (Figure 3). Given the larger surface are of the soles, 150 U of BoNT-ONA diluted in 6 to 8 mL of normal saline is injected in the same grid distribution using the same technique (Figure 4). Post-injection, ice packs are reapplied while the patient waits in the exam room for 15 minutes to further assist with pain and to confirm no immediate reaction to the toxin.

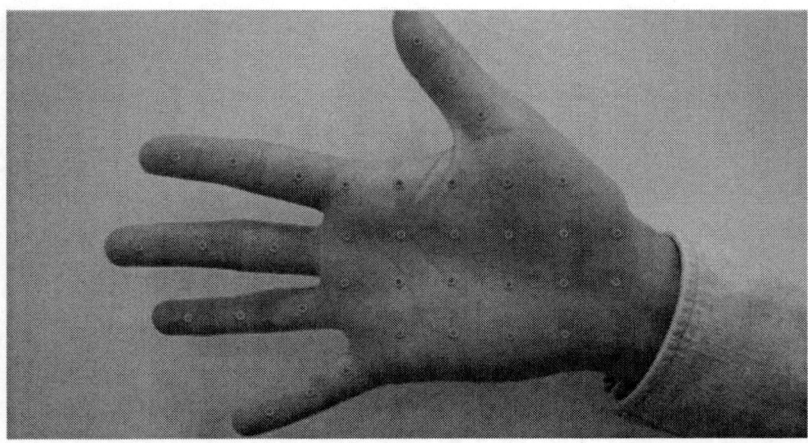

Figure 3. Injection grid for palmar hyperhidrosis.

Recently, a needle free approach to treating palmoplantar hyperhidrosis has been proposed using the MED-JET device (Medical International Technologies, Inc., Quebec, Canada), which uses a high-pressure spurt to deliver BoNT-ONA to the desired area. [50] Though the treatment may be optimal for the needle-phobic or apprehensive patient, the dose administered

(2 U/spurt) is greater than what is often desired, and further research must be conducted to evaluate the efficacy of the technique. [50, 51]

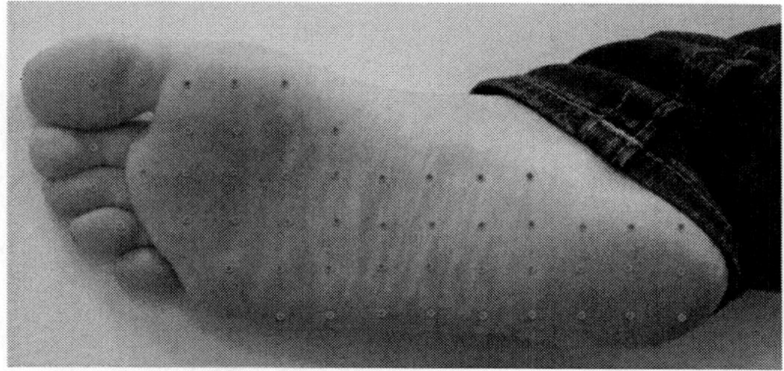

Figure 4. Injection grid for plantar hyperhidrosis.

Craniofacial Treatment

Focal hyperhidrosis of the face is often secondary to endocrine causes or pharmacologic side effects, making diagnosis of primary disease difficult. However, there are four major patterns of primary focal craniofacial hyperhidrosis, including symptoms in conjunction with ophiasis, a form of alopecia areata; diffuse or whole scalp; upper lip; and Frey syndrome (gustatory hyperhidrosis post-paradoidectomy). [52] Studies have suggested that BoNT-ONA can be effective in treatment; however, findings have been limited to case reports. The major issue with administering botulinum toxin to the facial region is aesthetic concerns, including facial asymmetry or brow ptosis. [53] Currently there is no consensus on the appropriate dosage, technique, or indications for using botulinum toxin for the treatment of craniofacial hyperhidrosis. [52-55]

Post-Treatment Care

The primary concern immediately after treatment is for an acute reaction to the injection. Patients are monitored in the office for signs and symptoms of adverse events post-treatment and are encouraged to report any adverse events that occur following treatments and between follow-up visits. Within two weeks of treatment, we routinely call patients to confirm they have begun to experience relief from their symptoms. Patients usually return for repeat treatment when their symptoms begin to recur.

Expected Outcomes

Efficacy and Duration of Effects

Improvement in symptoms can be detected within the first week after treatment for most patients. Rarely do patients experience initial treatment failure requiring reinjection with toxin. In our experience and as reported in the literature, botulinum toxin treatment for hyperhidrosis has an average duration of effect from six to nine months. [14, 24, 33] As the neurotoxin irreversibly reduces all acetylcholine transmission to the eccrine glands, we have observed that both moderate and severe cases of hyperhidrosis resolve equally with treatment. Interestingly for palmar hyperhidrosis specifically, a greater relief of symptoms has been observed in the non-dominant hand. Nevertheless, symptomatic relief and satisfaction are both reported amongst patients. [56]

Patient Satisfaction and Quality of Life

For many patients, the greatest challenge of hyperhidrosis is the detrimental effect of symptoms on quality of life (QoL) issues. In a 2002 multicenter, randomized, double-blind, placebo-controlled trial, the authors reported BoNT-ONA treatment of patients with primary axillary hyperhidrosis was associated with statistically significant improvement in the following categories: satisfaction with treatment compared to other previously attempted regimens, number of clothing changes per day, ability to participate in daily and social activities, professional productivity at work, and overall emotional status. [2]

In addition to the positive effect on QoL, treatment with botulinum toxin is also associated with a 63 percent increase in patient satisfaction in randomized placebo-controlled trials. [57] Additionally, patients prefer botulinum toxin over nonsurgical treatment options such as topical agents. [2, 22] In our experience, we have found that the majority of patients experience at least a 2-point improvement in HDSS score and report a satisfaction rate between 66% and 100%, confirming that patients are overall very happy with the treatment. [14, 24]

Natural History of the Disease

Primary hyperhidrosis is a chronic condition; in our experience, we have not seen patients experience permanent resolution of symptoms with treatment. Due to the effectiveness of treatment, however, we have found that patients are committed to receiving repeated injections over a number of years. [24] Nevertheless, there are also patients who only undergo one treatment session. This may be due to the expense of treatment or the discomfort associated with injections. [14, 24]

Adverse Effects

In addition to pain and discomfort at the time of injection, the most commonly published adverse complication associated with botulinum toxin injection is local muscle weakness, particularly in palmar disease. Weakness is usually observed on maximal opposition and is often transient, lasting for a few weeks after injection. [14, 58] Furthermore, in a study of 36 patients who underwent palmar treatment, one-third experienced marginal improvement of their plantar disease whereas two-thirds experienced statistically significant worsening of plantar hyperhidrosis as determined by gravimetry. [59] These findings may be due to a compensatory increase in systemic eccrine stimulation in response to local inactivation of acetylcholine receptors. More studies, however, will be needed to confirm these observations.

Disadvantages

The primary disadvantage of botulinum toxin in the treatment of hyperhidrosis is its impermanence, with symptomatic relief lasting typically from six to nine months. We found that patients who underwent more than four treatments for axillary disease tended to return more frequently for subsequent injections. [14, 24] For palmar disease, however, one study reported a statistically significant increase in duration of treatment effect from

7 to 9.5 months with repeated injections. [60] Some patients may develop antibodies to the toxin, reducing efficacy of treatment over time. [61] However we hypothesize that for axillary disease, patients may be less tolerant to symptoms after becoming accustomed to anhidrosis, causing them to seek repeated treatment more frequently.

Conclusion

Botulinum toxin type A injection is a safe, effective, and relatively long-lasting treatment option for symptomatic axillary, palmar, and plantar hyperhidrosis. Patients with craniofacial hyperhidrosis may also benefit from treatment. Ideal patients are those with moderate-to-severe hyperhidrosis, seasonal disease, or focal hyperhidrosis who seek excellent treatment results through a non-invasive procedure. Throughout the literature, patients report a high satisfaction rate with treatment, as well as an improvement in overall quality of life. Botulinum toxin therefore should be offered as a long-term management option for patients suffering from hyperhidrosis.

References

[1] Strutton, DR; Kowalski, JW; Glaser, DA; Stang, PE. US prevalence of hyperhidrosis and impact on individuals with axillary hyperhidrosis: results from a national survey. *J Am Acad Dermatol* 2004;51:241-248.

[2] Naumann, MK; Hamm, H; Lowe, NJ; on behalf of the Botox Hyperhidrosis Clinical Study Group. Effect of botulinum toxin type A on quality of life measures in patients with excessive axillary sweating: a randomized controlled trial. *Br J Dermatol* 2002;147:1218-1226.

[3] Solish, N; Benohanian, A; Kowalski, JW. Prospective open-label study of botulinum toxin type A in patients with primary axillary hyperhidrosis: effects on functional impairment and quality of life. *Dermatol Surg* 2005;31:405-413.

[4] Swartling, C; Naver, H; Lindberg, M. Botulinum A toxin improves life quality in severe primary focal hyperhidrosis. *Eur J Neurol* 2001;8:247-252.

[5] Campanati, A; Penna, L; Guzzo, T; Menotta, L; Silvestri, B; Lagalla, G; Gesuita, R; Offidani, A. Quality-of-life assessment in patients with

hyperhidrosis before and after treatment with botulinum toxin: results of an openlabel study. *Clin Ther* 2003;25:298-308.

[6] Hornberger, J; Grimes, K; Naumann, M; Glaser, DA; Lowe, NJ; Naver, H; Stolman, LP; Multi-Specialty Working Group on the Recognition, Diagnosis, and Treatment of Primary Focal Hyperhidrosis. Multispecialty working group on the recognition, diagnosis, and treatment of primary focal hyperhidrosis: recognition, diagnosis, and treatment of primary focal hyperhidrosis. *J Am Acad Dermatol* 2004;51:274-286.

[7] Zacherl, J; Huber, ER; Imhof, M; Plas, EG; Herbst, F; Függer, R. Long-term results of 630 thoracoscopic sympathicotomies for primary hyperhidrosis: the Vienna experience. *Eur J Surg Suppl* 1998;580:43-46.

[8] Lin, T; Wang, N; Huang, L. Pitfalls and complication avoidance associated with transthoracic endoscopic sympathectomy for primary hyperhidrosis (analysis of 2200 cases). *Int J Surg Investig* 2001;2:377-385.

[9] Gossot, D; Galetta, D; Pascal, A; Debrosse, D; Caliandro, R; Girard, P; Stern, JB; Grunewald, D. Long-term results of endoscopic thoracic sympathectomy for upper limb hyperhidrosis. *Ann Thorac Surg* 2003;75:1075-1079.

[10] Arneja, JS; Hayakawa, TEJ; Singh, GB; Murray, KA; Turner, RB; Ross, LL; Bendor-Samuel, RL. Axillary hyperhidrosis: a 5-year review of treatment efficacy and recurrence rates using a new arthroscopic shaver technique. *Plast Reconstr Surg* 2007;119:562-567.

[11] Tung, T. Endoscopic shaver with liposuction for treatment of axillary osmidrosis. *Ann Plast Surg* 2001;46:400-404.

[12] Flanagan, KH; King, R; Glaser, DA. Botulinum toxin type A versus topical 20% aluminum chloride for the treatment of moderate to severe primary focal axillary hyperhidrosis. *J Drugs Dermatol* 2008;7:221-227.

[13] Woolery-Lloyd, H; Valins, W. Aluminum chloride hexahydrate in a salicylic acid gel: a novel topical agent for hyperhidrosis with decreased irritation. *J Clin Aesthetic Dermatol* 2009;2:28-31.

[14] Doft, MA; Hardy, KL; Ascherman, JA. Treatment of Hyperhidrosis with Botulinum Toxin. *Aesthet Surg J* 2012;32(2):238-244.

[15] Bushara, KO; Park, DM; Jones, JC; Schutta, HS. Botulinum toxin—a possible new treatment for axillary hyperhidrosis. *Clin Exp Dermatol* 1996;21:276-278.

[16] Swartling, C; Naver, H; Pihl-Lundin, I; Hagforsen, E; Vahlquist, A. Sweat gland morphology and periglandular innervation in essential

palmar hyperhidrosis before and after treatment with intradermal botulinum toxin. *J Am Acad Dermatol* 2004;54:739-745.

[17] Glogau, RG. Botulinum A neurotoxin for axillary hyperhidrosis: no sweat Botox. *Dermatol Surg* 1998;24:817-819.

[18] Naver, H; Swartling, C; Aquilonius, SM. Palmar and axillary hyperhidrosis treated with botulinum toxin: one-year clinical follow-up. *Eur J Neurol* 2000;7:55-62.

[19] Naumann, M; Lowe, NJ. Botulinum toxin type A in treatment of bilateral primary axillary hyperhidrosis: randomized, parallel group, double blind, placebo-controlled trial. *Br Med J* 2001;323:596-599.

[20] Odderson, IR. Long-term quantitative benefits of botulinum toxin type A in the treatment of axillary hyperhidrosis. *Dermatol Surg* 2002;28:480-483.

[21] Heckmann, M; Ceballos-Baumann, AO; Plewig, G; Hyperhidrosis Study Group. Botulinum toxin A for axillary hyperhidrosis (excessive sweating). *N Engl J Med* 2001;344:488-493.

[22] Lowe, NJ; Glaser, DE; Eadie, N; Daggett, S; Kowalski, JW; Lai, PY; North American Botox in Primary Axillary Hyperhidrosis Clinical Study Group. Botulinum toxin type A in the treatment of primary axillary hyperhidrosis: a 52-week multicenter double-blind, randomized, placebo-controlled study of efficacy and safety. *J Am Acad Dermatol* 2007;56:604-611.

[23] Lowe, NJ. The place of botulinum toxin type A in the treatment of focal hyperhidrosis. *Br J Dermatol* 2004;151:1115-1122.

[24] Doft, M; Kasten, J; Ascherman, J. Treatment of axillary hyperhidrosis with botulinum toxin, a single surgeon's experience with 53 consecutive patients. *Aesthetic Plastic Surg* 2011;35:1079-1086.

[25] Lakraj, AAD; Moghimi, N; Jabbari, B. Hyperhidrosis: Anatomy, Pathophysiology and Treatment with Emphaisis on the Role of Botulinum Toxins. *Toxins* 2013;5:821-840.

[26] Basciani, M; Di Rienzo, F; Bizzarrini, M; Sanchi, M; Copetti, M; Intiso, D. Efficacy of botulinum toxin type B for the treatment of primary palmar hyperhidrosis: a prospective, open, single-blind, multi-centre study. *Arch Dermatol Res* 2014; Epub ahead of print (PMID: 24522897).

[27] Kariqvist, M; Rosell, K; Rystedt, A; Hymnelius, K; Swartling, C. Botulinum toxin B in the treatment of craniofacial hyperhidrosis. *J Eur Acad Dermatol Venereol* 2013; Epub ahead of print (PMID: 24118460).

[28] Atkins, JL; Butler, PEM. Hyperhidrosis: a review of current management. *Plast Reconstr Surg* 2002;110:222-228.

[29] Rompel, R; Scholz, S. Subcutaneous curettage vs. injection of botulinum toxin A for treatment of axillary hyperhidrosis. *J Eur Acad Dermatol Venereol* 2001;15:207-211.

[30] Vorkamp, T; Foo, F; Khan, S; Schmitto, JD; Wilson, P. Hyperhidrosis: evolving concepts and a comprehensive review. *Surgeon* 2010;8:287-292.

[31] Minor, V. Ein neues Verfahren zu der klinischen Untersuchung der Schweissabsonderung. *Deutche Zeitung Fürr Nervenheilkunde* 1928;101:302-308.

[32] Stefaniak, TJ; Procsko, M. Gravimetry in sweating assessment in primary hyperhidrosis and healthy individuals. *Clin Auton Res* 2013;23:197-200.

[33] Finlay, AY. Quality of life measurement in dermatology: a practical guide. *Br J Dermatol* 1997;136:305e14.

[34] Benson, RA; Palin, R; Holt, PJE; Loftus, IM. Diagnosis and management of hyperhidrosis. *BMJ* 2013;347:f6800 doi: 10.1136/bmj.f6800.

[35] Kowalski, JW; Eadie, N; Daggett, S; et al. Validity and reliability of the Hyperhidrosis Disease Severity Scale (HDSS). Poster presented at the 62nd Annual Meeting of the American Academy of Dermatology; February 6-10, 2004; Washington, DC. Poster P198.

[36] Bouman, H. The treatment of hyperhidrosis of hands and feet with constant current. *Am J Phys Med* 1952;31:158-169.

[37] Solish, N; Bertucci, V; Dansereau, A; Hong, HCH; Lynde, C; Lupin, M; Smith, KC; Storwick, G. A Comprehensive Approach to the Recognition, Diagnosis, and Severity-Based Treatment of Focal Hyperhidrosis: Recommendations of the Canadian Hyperhidrosis Advisory Committee. *Dermatol Surg* 2007;33:908-923.

[38] Kreyden, OP; Scheidegger, EP. Anatomy of the sweat glands, pharmacology of botulinum toxin, and distinctive syndromes associated with hyperhidrosis. *Clinic Derm* 2004;22:40-44.

[39] Farrugia, MK; Nicholls, EA. Intradermal botulinum A toxin injection for axillary hyperhidrosis. *J Pediatr Surg* 2005;40:1668-1669.

[40] Campanati, A; Giuliodori, K; Martina, E; Giulano, A; Ganzetti, G; Offidani, A. Onabotulinumtoxin type A (Botox (®)) versus Incobotulinumtoxin type A (Xeomin (®)) in the treatment of focal idiopathic palmar hyperhidrosis: results of a comparative double-blind clinical trial. *J Neural Transm* 2014;121(1):21-6.

[41] Brashear, A; Lew, MF; Dykstra, DD; Comella, CL; Factor, SA; Rodnitzky, RL; Trosch, R; Singer, C; Brin, MF; Murray, JJ; Wallace, JD; Willmer-Hulme, A; Koller, M. Safety and efficacy of Neurobloc (botulinum toxin type B) in type-A-responsive cervical dystonia. *Neurology* 1999;53:1439-1446.

[42] Basciani, M; Di Rienzo, F; Bizzarrini, M; Zanchi, M; Copetti, M; Intiso, D. Efficacy of botulinum toxin type B for the treatment of primary palmar hyperhidrosis: a prospective, open, single-blinded, multi-centre study. *Arch Dermatol Res* 2014; Epub ahead of print (PMID 24522897).

[43] Baumann, L; Slezinger, A; Halem, M; Vujevich, J; Martin, LK; Black, L; Bryde, J. Pilot study of the safety and efficacy of Myoblock (botulinum toxin type B) for the treatment of axillary hyperhidrosis. *Int J Dermatol* 2005;44(5):418-424.

[44] Frasson, E; Brigo, F; Acler, M; Didone, G; Vicentini, S; Bertolasi, L. Botulinum toxin type A vs type B for axillary hyperhidrosis in a case series of patients observed for 6 months. *Arch Dermatol* 2011;147(1):122-123.

[45] Dressler, D; Eleopra, R. Clinical use of non-A botulinum toxins: botulinum toxin type B. *Neurotox Res* 2006;9(2-3):121-125.

[46] Gülec, AT. Dilution of botulinum toxin A in lidocaine vs. in normal saline for the treatment of primary axillary hyperhidrosis: a double-blind, randomized, comparative preliminary study. *J Eur Acad Dermatol Venereol* 2011;26(3):314-318.

[47] Baumann, L; Frankel, S; Welsh, E; Halem, M. Cryoanalgesia with dichlorotetrafluoroethane lessens the pain of botulinum toxin injections for the treatment of palmar hyperhidrosis. *Dermatol Surg* 2003;29:1057e9.

[48] Benohanian, A. Needle-free anaesthesia prior to botulinum toxin type A injection treatment of palmar and plantar hyperhidrosis. *Br J Dermatol* 2007;156:593-596.

[49] Smith, K. Ice minimizes discomfort associated with injection of botulinum toxin type A for the treatment of palmar and plantar hyperhidrosis. *Dermatol Surg* 2007;33:S88-S91.

[50] Campanati, A; Giuliodori, K; Giuliano, A; Martina, E; Ganzetti, G; Marconi, B; Chiarici, A; Offidani, A. Treatment of palmar hyperhidrosis with botulinum toxin type A: results from a pilot study based on a novel injective approach. *Arch Dermatol Res* 2013;305:691-697.

[51] Patakfalvi, L; Benohanian, A. Treatment of palmar hyperhidrosis with needle-free injection of botulinum toxin A. *Arch Dermatol Res* 2014;306:101-102.

[52] George, SMC; Atkinson, LR; Farrant, PBJ; Shergill, BS. Botulinum toxin for focal hyperhidrosis of the face. *Br J Dermatol* 2014;170:211-213.

[53] Glaser, DA; Hebert, AA; Pariser, DM; Solish, N. Facial hyperhidrosis: best practice recommendations and special considerations. *Cutis* 2007;79(5 Suppl):29-32.

[54] Böger, A; Herath, H; Rompel, R; Ferbert, A. Botulinum toxin for treatment of craniofacial hyperhidrosis. *J Neurol* 2000;415:857-861.

[55] Santana-Rodriguez, N; Clavo-Varas, B; Ponce-González, MÁ; Jarabo-Sarceda, JR; Perez-Alonso, D; Ruiz Caballero, JA; Olmo-Quintana, V; Atallah Yordi, N; Fiuza-Pérez, MD. Primary frontal hyperhidrosis successfully treated with low doses of botulinum toxin A as a useful alternative to surgical treatment. *J Dermatolog Treat* 2012;23(1):49-51.

[56] Solomon, BA; Hayman, R. Botulinum toxin type A therapy for palmar and digital hyperhidrosis. *J Am Acad Dermatol* 2000;42:1026-1029.

[57] Naumann, M; Lowe, NJ; Kumar, CR; Hamm, H; Hyperhidrosis Clinical Investigators Group. Botulinum toxin type A is a safe and effective treatment for axillary hyperhidrosis over 16 months: a prospective study. *Arch Dermatol* 2003;139:731-736.

[58] Glaser, DA; Hebert, AA; Pariser, DM; Solish, N. Palmar and plantar hyperhidrosis: best practice recommendations and special considerations. *Cutis* 2007;79(suppl 5):18-28.

[59] Gregoriou, S; Rigopoulos, D; Makris, M; Liakou, A; Agiosofitou, E; Stefanaki, C; Kontochristopoulos, G. Effects of Botulinum Toxin-A Therapy for Palmar Hyperhidrosis in Plantar Sweat Production. *Dermatol Surg* 2010;36:496-498.

[60] Lecouflet, M; Leux, C; Fenot, M; Célerier, P; Maillard, H. Duration of efficacy increases with the repetition of botulinum toxin A injections in primary palmar hyperhidrosis: A study of 28 patients. *J Am Acad Dermatol* 2014; Epub ahead of print (PMID: 24630001).

[61] Boni, R; Kreyden, OP; Burg, G. Revival of the use of botulinum toxin: application in dermatology. *Dermatology* 2000;200:287-291.

In: Hyperhidrosis
Editor: Janine R. Huddle

ISBN: 978-1-63321-516-0

Chapter II

Physiopathology of Hyperhidrosis

Nabor Bezerra de Moura Júnior*
Federal University of Piaui, Teresina, Brazil

Abstract

The physiopathology of primary hyperhidrosis is not completely understood: eccrine sweat glands are normal in number, size, and function in hyperhidrotic patients. Nevertheless, such patients show abnormal sympathetic skin response, suggesting that the cause of hyperhidrosis may be related to a sympathetic nervous system (which innervates eccrine sweat glands) dysfunction. Despite the resection of thoracic sympathetic chain ganglia be a treatment for primary hyperhidrosis, the function of sympathetic ganglia in normal individuals and in hyperhidrotic patients remained unknown until a short time ago. Our studies showed abnormalities in size, ganglion cells count, collagen fibers (using picrosirius staining)/elastic fibers (using Weigert's resorcin-fuchsin method) ratio, apoptosis (using caspase-3 assay), expression of acetylcholine, and expression of a specific subunit of nicotinic acetylcholine receptor in sympathetic ganglia of hyperhidrotic patients. Such results confirm the premise that sympathetic ganglia play an

* Email: nabor@usp.br.

important role in the pathophysiology of primary hyperhidrosis and may indicate new treatment modalities for this condition.

Sweating is a physiological process responsible for regulating body temperature. It increases during exercise, excessive heat, or stressful situations. [1-6] Hyperhidrosis is defined as excessive sweating of the eccrine glands in nonphysiological conditions and may be generalized or focal, affecting mainly the palms, soles, armpits, and face. [1-4, 6, 7]

Occasionally, there is an underlying etiology, which justifies hyperhidrosis. However, in many people, excessive sweating occurs in the absence of other conditions that justify it, when it is classified as primary hyperhidrosis (PH). [1-3, 8]

Its prevalence may reach 2.8% of the population and affects both genders similarly and in all age groups, varying only the age of onset of symptoms according to the most affected part of the body: childhood for palmar and plantar hyperhidrosis, adolescence for axillary hyperhidrosis, and adulthood for craniofacial hyperhidrosis. There is a family history associated with PH between 12.5% and 56.5% of patients, according to epidemiological studies. [1, 9, 10]

The physiopathology of PH is not well understood. Morphological studies in the sweat glands of patients with PH showed no change in their number or histology. [2, 3, 5-7, 11, 12]

The sweat glands are innervated in a quite particular way: by cholinergic fibers of the sympathetic nervous system, and they also do not have parasympathetic innervation, although they are related to hypothalamic nuclei considered parasympathetic. [6, 7, 13-16]; it is believed that a complex dysfunction of the autonomic nervous system (ANS) is related to its etiology.

1. Sympathetic Activity and Hyperhidrosis

Hyperhidrotic patients have overactive sympathetic nervous system, demonstrated by the sympathetic skin response. At the same time, the change in skin blood flow following the variation of the temperature was similar to normal individuals (which decreases after sympathectomy), suggesting that despite being part of the thermoregulatory system, sweat glands and blood vessels receive innervation from distinct groups of sympathetic fibers. [5, 12, 17-20]

Treatment of moderate/severe cases of PH is based on medical or surgical blockade of sympathetic stimulation, whether it is local (e.g., using botulinum toxin A) or systemic (e.g., using oxybutynin); endoscopic resection of one or more ganglia of the thoracic sympathetic chain is constituted today as the most efficient palmar, axillary, and craniofacial control method of PH, especially for the former. [1, 2, 8, 11, 21, 22]

Therefore, a proper understanding of the physiopathology of PH must pass through the study of the functional aspects of the anatomical structures that make up the autonomic nervous system.

1.1. Sympathetic Skin Response

Sympathetic activity in a certain part of the body can be estimated by measuring the skin resistance to electrical conduction, an indirect measure of sympathetic sudomotor function. Previous studies have shown elevated sympathetic skin response (latency, duration, and peak amplitude) in patients with PH compared with healthy individuals, although some authors have found it next to normal. To clarify the question, the excitability recovery curve of the sympathetic skin response (duration of refractoriness to a second electrical stimulus after administration of an initial stimulus), more reliable, was analyzed. It confirmed the finding of hyperactivity of the sympathetic system in patients with PH. [5, 12, 17, 23, 24]

1.2. Heart Rate Variability

The heart rate variability (HRV) brings us information about the sympathetic/parasympathetic balance over the heart. However, several studies of the spectral analysis of HRV have shown quite different results in PH patients: low frequencies of heart rate variability (the Valsalva maneuvers and immersing the face in cold water) compared with normal subjects, which rises to normal levels after sympathectomy. [25-27] These patients seem to present a higher parasympathetic tonus than the controls. [16] It was also noted that sympathectomy reduces the heart rate during rest and orthostatic stress because of an increased parasympathetic and reduced sympathetic activity, without significant change in cardiopulmonary exercise testing. Although there are no studies to date that could prove it, this finding may be beneficial to individuals with high levels of sympathetic activity; once, this may be deleterious. [26-28]

1.3. Postural Hypotension

Hyperhidrotic patients show higher decreases in blood pressure values during orthostatism and tilt test at 65°. Such finding may be related to a possible dysfunction in the ANS or due to a dehydration caused by a higher water loss. [16]

1.4. Blood Pressure

Patients with PH show a greater increase in blood pressure during tilt-test than the controls. After sympathectomy, these values tend to normalize, being similar to that of healthy individuals. [26]

1.5. Baroreceptor Sensitivity

Sympathectomy induces a higher baroreceptor sensitivity, when compared with values of both preoperative and the normal subjects. This finding also suggests a proportionally increased parasympathetic tonus in such patients. [26]

2. Anatomy and Physiology of the Autonomic Nervous System

The autonomic or visceral efferent nervous system is the portion of the nervous system responsible for homeostasis and, therefore, the regulation of body temperature, among others. [29] Its operation is independent of the will of the individual, whence its name. Anatomically, it is formed by neurons and preganglionic and postganglionic fibers; the former is located in the brainstem, where some cranial nerves originate, and the latter is located in the spinal cord from the first thoracic segment to the fourth sacral segment, forming a part of the gray matter known as lateral column of spinal cord in its thoracolumbar portion. [30, 31]

The cell bodies of postganglionic neurons are concentrated outside the central nervous system (CNS), forming the ganglia. In these cell bodies (perikarya), one can visualize rough endoplasmic reticulum associated with free polyribosomes in large numbers, forming the so-called Nissl bodies, whose amount varies according to the functional state of the neuron. [30-32]

Connections of preganglionic neurons with the limbic system, particularly the hypothalamus, may justify the interdependence of emotions with its function, producing, for example, profuse palmar sweating under stress, even in person without hyperhidrosis. [30, 31, 33, 34]

The autonomic nervous system is classically divided in sympathetic and parasympathetic systems. At first, the preganglionic neurons are located in the lateral column of the thoracolumbar spinal cord, and the postganglionic ganglia form the prevertebral and paravertebral sympathetic chain, a structure formed by many ganglia and their respective interganglionares branches extending from the region posterior cervical, on each side, to the coccyx, where the two chains are fused together.

The parasympathetic preganglionic neurons are located in the brainstem and the sacral cord, whereas the postganglionic neurons are located near or within the effector organ. [30, 31]

Functionally, the sympathetic postganglionic fibers are characterized by the production of noradrenaline (noradrenergic fibers or simply adrenergic), whereas the parasympathetic produce acetylcholine (cholinergic fibers) to produce antagonistic effects on most of the effector organs. The preganglionic fibers, on the other hand, are both cholinergic for sympathetic and parasympathetic nervous system. [16, 30]

In turn, the sweat glands are innervated by cholinergic postganglionic fibers, despite being part of the sympathetic system, in addition to not receiving parasympathetic innervation; the excitation of these fibers stimulates the production and excretion of sweat. Furthermore, hypothalamic centers related to perspiration are considered generally parasympathetic. [6, 16, 30]

The preganglionic sympathetic myelinated fibers that emerge from the lateral column of the cord through the ventral root forming the white communicating branches synapse with postganglionic spinal neuron, which in turn can be located in a paravertebral ganglion at the same level of the fiber, in a paraspinal ganglion located at levels above or below the level of the fiber (interganglionares branches forming the sympathetic chain) or in a prevertebral ganglion through the splanchnic nerves. From the ganglia, run the unmyelinated postganglionic fibers forming the gray communicating branch and head to the effector organ, associated or not to a spinal nerve. [30, 31]

Even before the actual knowledge of the autonomic nervous system, in the eighteenth century, Jacobus Benignus Winslow (1669-1760) suggested that the sympathetic chain ganglia would have spinal origin; so a brain-independent structure; ganglia would be independent "small brains". [41]

At the end of the same century, Marie François Xavier Bichat (1771-1802) proposed an anatomical and functional separation of life (and nervous system) in two forms: the "organic life", characterized by continuity, asymmetry, disharmony, and independence habits and education, would be commanded by the ganglia and would end with the death of the heart. On the other hand, the "animal life" would be characterized by discontinuity, symmetry, and harmony and influenced by the external environment, and this command would come from the brain and end with its death, which could happen before the death of many other organs; the sympathetic chain was not a nerve but a set of "small brains" (as proposed by Winslow), hence the name “ganglionic nervous system”. [41]

Since the anatomical characterization of the autonomic nervous system by Langley, it was believed that the sympathetic ganglion functioned only as a relay of an impulse generated in the central nervous system on its way to the effector organ; however, from the work of Eccles, it was realized that the autonomic ganglion has an active role in the modulation and distribution of this impulse, either by synapses themselves or excitatory or inhibitory postsynaptic potentials. [18 - 20] These recent studies confirm the hypothesis currently accepted: that the sympathetic ganglia modulate nervous stimuli from the CNS, with high concentrations of both acetylcholine as a specific lineage of its receptors, playing an important role in the pathophysiology of PH. At the same time, such studies reaffirmed the theories of "small brains" of Winslow and "organic life" of Bichat, while it demonstrated anatomical and functional alteration, producing localized autonomic ganglionic pathology. [18, 25, 41-44]

2.1. The Sympathetic Ganglia

Hyperhidrotic patients have bigger sympathetic ganglia, located in the thoracic sympathetic chain. This may not usually be noticed during operations because of the small difference found (less than 2 millimeters) that becomes significant because of the small size of the ganglia. [13]

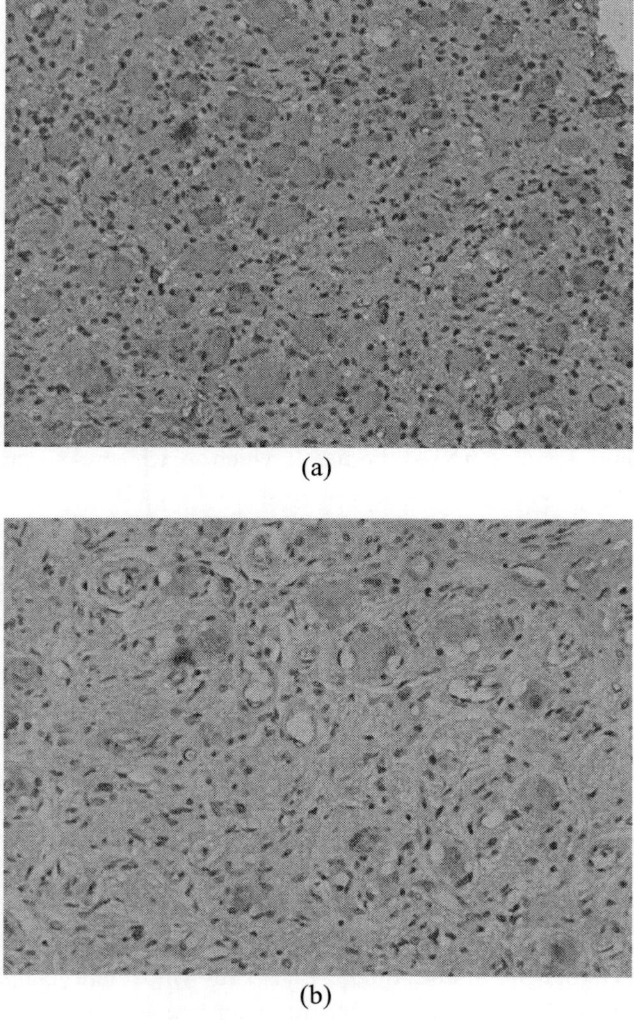

(a)

(b)

Figure 1. Expression of acetylcholine in the third thoracic sympathetic ganglion. A: Hyperhidrosis. B: Control.

They also show structural abnormalities in their ganglia, when compared with nonhyperhidrotic people. The former have more ganglion cells than was observed in the controls. Picrosirius staining also shows few collagen fibers in patients with hyperhidrosis. The opposite occurs in nonhyperhidrotic people: there is a lower number of ganglion cells and a larger area that contains collagen within the ganglion. [14]

Additionally, more ganglion cells in apoptosis were found in the ganglia of patients with hyperhidrosis using caspase-3 immunohistochemical staining. These findings suggest that there is a proportionally greater amount of ganglion cells in patients with hyperhidrosis, causing more apoptosis and less space to the extracellular matrix. [14]

Sympathetic ganglia of patients with PH present acetylcholine in quantities approximately three times higher than those in noncarriers, as seen in Figure 1. Such overexpression can be observed in both cell bodies and synaptic clefts. It may be related to the presence of hyperactivity of the central portion of the sympathetic nervous system (preganglionic neurons located in the lateral column of the spinal cord), releasing a large amount of the neurotransmitter in the synaptic clefts existing in the ganglion or may be related to increased production of acetylcholine by the cell bodies of postganglionic neurons (Nissl bodies), which reach the sweat glands by anterograde flow from the perikarya to the axon. [13, 32]

However, because of the fact that both the area of strong expression of acetylcholine (coloring especially the Nissl bodies) as the area of weak expression of acetylcholine (diffuse expression, analogous to the distribution of synaptic clefts) in the sympathetic ganglion were increased, seems to demonstrate a combination of both events. [13]

2.2. Neuronal Nicotinic Acetylcholine Receptor

Acetylcholine exerts its role by binding to postsynaptic receptors, triggering an action potential that transmits the nerve impulse. These receptors can be classified as nicotinic or muscarinic according to the agonist molecule used to identify them; nicotinic receptors, in turn, are subdivided into neuronal and muscle (found in motor endplates). [15] In sympathetic ganglia, the type of acetylcholine receptor responsible for neurotransmission is the neuronal nicotinic (nAChR). [29, 35]

The nAChR is a transmembrane ion channel that, once activated by binding with acetylcholine, mediates fast synaptic transmission in sympathetic ganglia, formed by α and β subunits. In humans, these subunits are divided into several subtypes being recognized, eight α subunits (α2 - α7, α9, and α10) and three β (β2 - β4) between neuronal nicotinic receptors. The bond to the molecule agonists is made via two cysteine residues at the end of the α subunits, which differ them from the β subunits. [29, 35] The receptors are formed by a pentamer of two α and three β subunits in different combinations. As an exception, there are receptors formed only by α7 subunits.

Autonomic ganglia express the subunits α3, α4, α5, α7, β2, and β4, with a predominance of subunit α3, and prevailing compositions are the α3β4 and α3β2 heteromers, beyond the α7 homomer, although its distribution is not uniform across different ganglia, even different neurons in the same ganglion; the functional role of most of these receptors is still unclear. [18, 29, 35-38] The genes encoding these subunits have been identified: the 15q24 locus is responsible for subunits α3, α5, and β4, whereas the α7 subunit is encoded in the location 15q14, partially duplicated, which hinders their genetic analysis. [29]

2.2.1. The α3 Subunit

This subunit corresponds to the predominant subunit in the ganglia of the autonomic nervous system, most often associated with the β4 subunit, forming the receptor known as "ganglionic type." It is the main subunit responsible for the binding of the agonist to the receptor molecules, triggering synaptic transmission and presenting a significant proliferation in the development phase of the nervous system. [35-40]

Hyperhidrotic patients have similar amounts of α3 subunit, when compared with controls, despite the general alterations found in such sympathetic ganglia as size and ganglion cells count. Because this is the main subunit of the sympathetic ganglion, this finding may suggest a pathway mediated by a specific receptor. [15]

2.2.2. The α4 and α5 Subunits

While developing a crucial role in the CNS, the α4 subunit is rarely found in autonomic ganglia, with their presence in such structures being questioned for a long time. The α5 subunit plays a more structural role than binding to acetylcholine and is always associated with the α3 subunit in the sympathetic ganglia; their number does not vary significantly after birth. [18, 35, 38, 39]

2.2.3. The α7 Subunit

Although it may be associated with other α and β subunits, the main form of its expression takes the form of homomer, aberrant when compared with other receptors. It is characterized by rapid desensitization and high permeability to calcium and is vital in calcium-dependent events in the ganglion cells. It is located both in the presynaptic and in the postsynaptic membrane, modulating neurotransmitter release and regulating neuronal growth, and, as the α3 subunit, also provides a substantial increase in its number in the sympathetic ganglia during nervous system development. [35,38-40]

Immunohistochemical analysis of the sympathetic ganglia reveals that patients with PH express antibody against the α7 subunit of the neuronal nicotinic acetylcholine receptor more intensely than the controls (more than twice, as can be seen in Figure 02). [13]

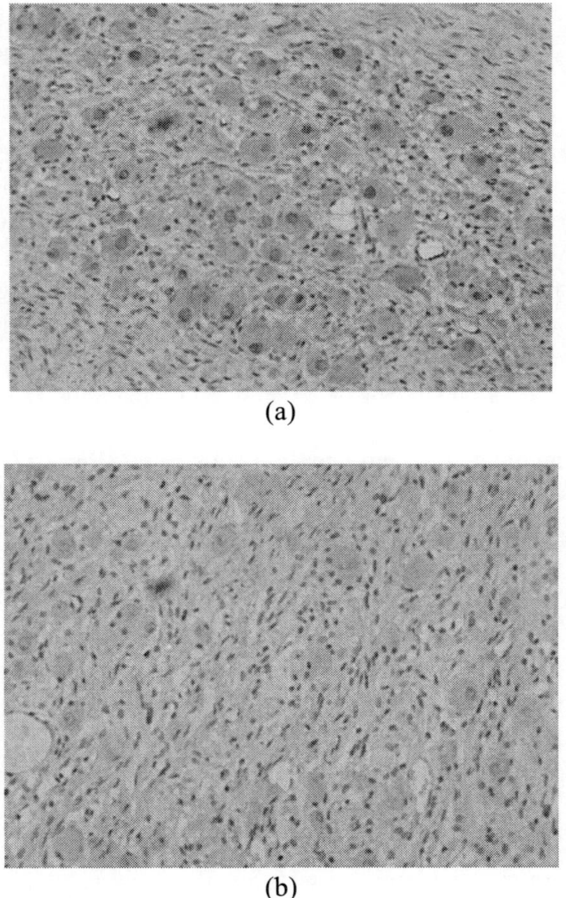

(a)

(b)

Figure 2. Expression of the α7 subunit of the nicotinic acetylcholine receptor in the third thoracic sympathetic ganglion. A: Hyperhidrosis. B: Control.

2.2.4. The β Subunits

Autonomic ganglia express the β2 and β4 subunits, always in association with α subunit, especially α3. As well as the α5 subunit, they also show no significant increase in their number during postnatal development. The specific blockade of one subunit is able to reduce the transmembrane currents to reach a plateau, but it is unable to abolish such currents completely, suggesting the involvement of multiple receptors with different conformations in the autonomic ganglia. [35, 38, 39]

3. The Role of the Central Nervous System

The autonomic nervous system has many interactions with the central nervous system. Some authors consider such structures as the central part of the ANS. It is believed that the main components are the nuclei tractus solitarii, the formatio reticularis, and the hypothalamus, although these associations are not fully understood. [33]

Sweat glands on the palms and soles have little thermoregulatory function and become active mainly by emotional stimuli. Some cortical projections to the hypothalamus (e.g., frontal and premotor) are believed to promote sweating during stressful situations. It is believed that these hypothalamic sweat centers are actually under exclusive control of the cortex, without influence from the thermoregulatory afferents. Thus, the emotional sweating stimulus should originate from the cerebral cortex (frontal and premotor areas) and reach the sweat glands passing through the hypothalamus, the lateral horn of the spinal cord and the sympathetic ganglia. Most of the sympathetic fibers arising from the hypothalamus cross at the level of the pons, and most of this crossing is completed in the medulla oblongata. [34]

Conclusion

Hyperhidrosis has a complex and not fully understood physiopathology. It is clear that hyperhidrotic patients show hyperactivation of the sympathetic nervous system and, probably, the parasympathetic system. It is also well defined that the sympathetic ganglia of patients with PH have structural and functional differences from noncarriers. Further studies must elucidate the effect and impact of the central nervous system in this disease.

References

[1] De Campos JRM, Kauffman P, Werebe EC, Andrade Filho LO, Kusniek S, Wolosker N, Jatene FB. Quality of life, before and after thoracic sympathectomy – report on 378 operated patients. *Ann. Thorac. Surg.*, 2003; 76:886 –91.

[2] Hornberger J, Grimes K, Naumann M, Glaser DA, Lowe NJ, Naver H, Ahn S, Stolman LP, Multi-Specialty Working Group on the Recognition, Diagnosis, and Treatment of Primary Focal Hyperhidrosis. Recognition, diagnosis and treatment of primary focal hyperhidrosis. *J. Am. Acad. Dermatol.*, 2004; 51:164-86.

[3] Eisenhach JH, Atkinson JLD, Fealey RD. Hyperhidrosis: evolving therapies for a well-established phenomenon. *Mayo Clin. Proc.*, 2005; 80(5):657-66.

[4] Wörle B, Rapprich S, Heckmann M. Definition and treatment of primary hyperhidrosis. *JDDG*, 2007; 7:325-8.

[5] Vetrugno R, Liguori R, Cortelli P, Montagna P. Sympathetic skin response: basical mechanisms and clinical applications. *Clin. Auton. Res.*, 2003; 13:256-70.

[6] Sato K, Kang WH, Saga K, Sato KT. Biology of sweat glands and their disorders I: normal sweat gland function. *J. Am. Acad. Dermatol.*, 1989; 20: 537-63.

[7] Sato K, Kang WH, Saga K, Sato KT. Biology of sweat glands and their disorders II: disorders of sweat gland function. *J. Am. Acad. Dermatol.*, 1989; 20: 713-15.

[8] Leung AKC, Chan PYH, Choi MCK. Hyperhidrosis. *Int. J. Dermatol.,* 1999; 38:561-7.

[9] Strutton DR, Kowalski JW, Glaser DA, Stang PE. US prevalence of hyperhidrosis and impact on individuals with axillary hyperhidrosis: results from a national survey. *J. Am. Acad. Dermatol.,* 2004; 51:241-8.

[10] Lear W, Kessler E, Solish N, Glaser DA. An epidemiological study of hyperhidrosis. *Dermatol Surg*. 2007; 33:S69-75.

[11] Wenzel FG, Horn TD. Nonneoplastic disorders of the eccrine glands. *J. Am. Acad. Dermatol.*, 1998; 38:1-17.

[12] Manca D, Valls-Solé J, Callejas MA. Excitability recovery curve of the sympathetic skin response in healthy volunteers and patients with palmar hyperhidrosis. *Clin. Neurophysiol.*, 2000; 111: 1767-70.

[13] de Moura Júnior NB, das-Neves-Pereira JC, de Oliveira FR, Jatene FB, Parra ER, Capelozzi VL, Wolosker N, de Campos JR. Expression of acetylcholine and its receptor in human sympathetic ganglia in primary hyperhidrosis. *Ann. Thorac. Surg.*, 2013;95(2):465-70.

[14] de Oliveira FR, Moura NB Jr, de Campos JR, Wolosker N, Parra ER, Capelozzi VL, Pêgo-Fernandes P. Morphometric Analysis of Thoracic Ganglion Neurons in Subjects with and without Primary Palmar Hyperhidrosis. *Ann. Vasc. Surg.*, 2014;28(4):1013-9.

[15] de Moura Júnior NB, das-Neves-Pereira JC, de Campos JR, de Oliveira FR, Wolosker N, Parra ER, Capelozzi VL, Jatene FB. Preservation of α-3 neuronal nicotinic acetylcholine receptor expression in sympathetic ganglia after brain death. *Mol. Neurobiol.*, 2012;45(2):362-5.

[16] De Marinis M, Colaizzo E, Petrelli RA, Santilli V. Alterations in cardiovascular autonomic function tests in idiopathic hyperhidrosis. *Auton. Neurosci.*, 2012;167(1-2):34-8.

[17] Kazemi B, Yahyaii L, Salmanpour R, Hadianfard MJ, Shirzi ZR. Comparison of sympathetic skin response between palmar hyperhidrotic and normal subjects. *Electromyogr. Clin. Neurophysiol.*, 2004; 44: 51-5.

[18] De Biasi M. Nicotinic mechanisms in the autonomic control of organ systems. *J. Neurobiol.*, 2002; 53:568-79.

[19] Bornmyr S, Svensson H, Söderström T, Sundkvist G, Wollmer P. Finger skin blood flow in response to indirect cooling in normal subjects and in patients before and after sympathectomy. *Clin. Physiol.*, 1998; 18: 103-7.

[20] Bini G, Hagbarth KE, Hynninen P, Wallin BG. Regional similarities and differences in thermoregulatory vaso- and sudomotor tone. *J. Physiol.*, 1980; 306: 553-65.

[21] De Campos JRM, Kauffman P. Video-assisted thoracic sympathectomy in the treatment of primary hyperhidrosis. *J. Bras. Pneumol.,* 2007; 33: xv-xvii.

[22] Krasna MJ. Thorachoscopic sympathectomy: a standardized approach to therapy for hyperhidrosis. *Ann. Thorac. Surg.* 2008; 85: S764-7.

[23] Chen HJ, Cheng MH, Lin TK, Chee EC. Recordings of pre- and postoperative sympathetic skin response in patients with palmar hyperhidrosis. *Stereotatic. Funct. Neurosurg.*, 1995; 64: 214-20.

[24] Lefaucheur JP, Fitoussi M, Becquemin JP. Abolition of sympathetic skin responses following endoscopic thoracic sympathectomy. *Muscle Nerve.*, 1996; 19: 581-6.

[25] Shih CJ, Wu JJ, Lin MT. Autonomic dysfunction in palmar hyperhidrosis. *J. Auton. Nerv. Syst.*, 1983; 8: 33-43.

[26] Bygstad E, Terkelsen AJ, Pilegaard HK, Hansen J, Mølgaard H, Hjortdal VE. Thoracoscopic sympathectomy increases efferent cardiac vagal activity and baroreceptor sensitivity. *Eur. J. Cardiothorac. Surg.*, 2013; 44 (3): e193-9.

[27] Cruz J, Sousa J, Oliveira AG, Silva-Carvalho L. Effects of endoscopic thoracic sympathectomy for primary hyperhidrosis on cardiac autonomic nervous activity. *J Thorac Cardiovasc Surg.* 2009;137:664–9.

[28] Noppen M, Vincken W. Thoracoscopic sympathicolysis for essential hyperhidrosis: effects on pulmonary function. *Eur. Respir. J*, 1996;9(8):1660-4.

[29] Kirstein SL, Insel PA. Autonomic nervous system pharmacogenomics: a progress report. *Pharmacol. Rev.*, 2004; 56: 31-52.

[30] Roosterman D1, Goerge T, Schneider SW, Bunnett NW, Steinhoff M. Neuronal control of skin function: the skin as a neuroimmunoendocrine organ. *Physiol. Rev.*, 2006; 86(4): 1309-79.

[31] McCormack AC1, Jarral OA, Shipolini AR, McCormack DJ. Does the nerve of Kuntz exist? *Interact. Cardiovasc. Thorac. Surg.*, 2011; 13(2): 175-8.

[32] Fletcher TF. Neurohistology atlas [cited 18 nov 2011]. Available at: http://vanat.cvm.umn.edu/neurHistAtls/pages/neuron7.html.

[33] Dressler D. Botulinum toxin therapy: its use for neurological disorders of the autonomic nervous system. *J. Neurol.,* 2013;150(3):701-13.

[34] Lakraj AA1, Moghimi N, Jabbari B. Hyperhidrosis: anatomy, pathophysiology and treatment with emphasis on the role of botulinum toxins. *Toxins*, 2013;5(4):821-40.

[35] Sargent PB. The diversity of neuronal nicotinic acetylcholine receptors. *Annu. Rev. Neurosci.*, 1993; 16: 403-43.

[36] Yeh JJ, Ferreira M, Ebert S, Yasuda RP, Kellar KJ, Wolfe BB. Axotomy and nerve growth factor regulate levels of neuronal nicotinic acetylcholine receptor α3 subunit protein in the rat superior cervical ganglion. *J. Neurochem.*, 2001; 79:258-65.

[37] Xu W, Gelber S, Orr-Urtreger A, Armstrong D, Lewis RA, Ou CN, Patrick J, Role L, De Biasi M, Beaudet AL. Megacystis, mydriasis, and

ion channel defect in mice lacking the α3 neuronal nicotinic acetylcholine receptor. *Neurobiology*, 1999; 96:5746-51.

[38] Skok VI. Nicotinic acetylcholine receptors in autonomic ganglia. *Auton. Neurosci.*, 2002; 97:1-11.

[39] Mandelzys A, Pié B, Deneris ES, Cooper E. The developmental increase in ACh current densities on rat sympathetic neurons correlates with changes in nicotinic ACh receptor α-subunit gene expression and occurs independent of innervation. *J. Neurosci.*, 1994; 14: 1357-64.

[40] Srivatsan M, Treece J, Shotts EE. Nicotine alters nicotinic receptor subunit levels differently in developing mammalian sympathetic neurons. *Ann. NY Acad. Sci.*, 2006; 1074: 505-13.

[41] Ackerknecht EH. The history of the discovery of the vegetative (autonomic) nervous system. *Med. Hist.*, 1974; 18: 1-8.

[42] Langley JN. On axon-reflexes in the pre-ganglionic fibres of the sympathetic system. *J. Physiol.*, 1900; 25: 364-98.

[43] Eccles JC. The action potential of the superior cervical ganglion. *J. Physiol.*, 1935; 85: 179-206.

[44] Eccles JC. Facilitation and inhibition in the superior cervical ganglion. *J. Physiol.*, 1935; 85: 207-38.

In: Hyperhidrosis
Editor: Janine R. Huddle
ISBN: 978-1-63321-516-0

Chapter III

Minimally Invasive Thoracoscopic Sympathectomy

Simon C. Y. Chow[1], M.B.Ch.B., M.R.C.S. and Calvin S. H. Ng[2*], B.Sc.(Hons), M.B.B.S.(Hons)(Lon), M.D.(Lon), F.R.C.S.Ed.(CTh)

[1]Senior Resident, Division of Cardiothoracic Surgery, The Chinese University of Hong Kong, Prince of Wales Hospital, Shatin, N.T., Hong Kong SAR, China

[2]Associate Professor, Department of Surgery, The Chinese University of Hong Kong, Prince of Wales Hospital, Shatin, N.T., Hong Kong SAR, China

Abstract

Hyperhidrosis can be a debilitating condition that affects patient's quality of life. Despite numerous non-surgical alternatives in the treatment algorithm, division of thoracic sympathetic nerves by surgery remains the most definitive treatment option and provides long-lasting

* Correspondence: Calvin S.H. Ng, BSc(Hons) MBBS(Hons) MD FRCSEd(CTh) Division of Cardiothoracic Surgery, The Chinese University of Hong Kong; Prince of Wales Hospital, Shatin, N.T. Hong Kong SAR, China; E-mail: calvinng@surgery.cuhk.edu.hk; Tel.No.: (852) 2632 2629Fax No.: (852) 2637 7974.

results. The history of surgical sympathectomy goes back several decades, however, the access trauma of thoracotomy was a significant drawback and the main resistance to the popularization of the procedure. The invention of thoracoscopes and subsequently the development of minimal invasive thoracoscopic sympathectomy saw the increasing acceptance of the technique by patients for treatment of hyperhidrosis. The last decade has seen the surgery evolving from 3-ports to single port access, and use of 10mm thoracoscopes and instruments to the needlescopic 3mm wide instruments, which improve aesthetics and patient satisfaction with promising therapeutic results. The development of embryonic natural orifice transluminal endoscopic surgery (E-NOTES) thoracic sympathectomy holds promise in further reducing access trauma. Despite the emergence of new minimally invasive techniques, many questions concerning surgical sympathectomy remain unanswered. Issues including the level at which sympathetic interruption should occur, and how the interruption should be achieved (sympathectomy, sympathicotomy or clipping) are explored in this chapter. Furthermore, we are only just beginning to understand the undesirable effects of thoracic sympathectomy and potential surgical remedies available. The chapter will review the available literature, and share the authors' experiences on these important issues relating to thoracoscopic sympathectomy.

Keywords: needlescopic, robotic, sympathectomy, uniport, videothoracoscopy

Introduction

Primary hyperhidrosis (PH) is a disorder of eccrine glands. Patients experience excessive sweating greater than physiological needs for thermoregulation. PH can be a debilitating condition, which affects quality of life as well as leads to feelings of shame and low self-esteem. The incidence of PH is quoted to be 1-3 %, with prevalence of 4-5% in western countries and Eastern populations alike. [1, 2, 3] The condition mostly affects young adults with onset during puberty and has no predilection for male or female. A family history of PH is not uncommon. Characteristic pattern of PH is usually focal, symmetrical and commonly precipitated by emotional and environmental triggers. Night sweating is very rare. PH commonly affects the palms and axilla, followed by the soles, and craniofacial region. The cause of PH remains unclear, with postulations suggesting that it may be related to over activity of the central nervous system and over stimulation of the eccrine glands. Eccrine glands are innervated by the sympathetic nerve fibers with acetylcholine being the major neurotransmitter; hence therapeutic targets are developed based on this understanding.

Treatment of PH can be categorized into non-surgical and surgical options. Non-surgical treatment includes the use of oral (for example, propantheline and oxybutynin) or topical medications (for example, aluminum chloride and glycopyrrolate), iontophoresis and botulinum toxin. The efficacy of nonsurgical treatment for PH is unpredictable and modest. Treatments such as iontophoresis and botulinum toxin injections require long term maintenance therapy for sustained effect, and recurrences are common. Lifelong treatment is also less cost effective when compared to surgery, especially in patients with severe hyperhidrosis.

Thoracic sympathectomy was first reported in 1920 by Kotzareff. [4] The aim was to achieve permanent relief in patients with medically refractory PH. Sympathectomy was not popularized until Kux reported the thoracoscopic approach for sympathectomy which significantly reduced access trauma, and made sympathectomy more acceptable amongst patients. [5] Formally introduced in the 1980s, endoscopic thoracic sympathectomy (ETS) has become the mainstay treatment for severe cases of PH. Over the past 20 years, there have been substantial improvements in endoscopic techniques and major advances in minimal invasive surgical equipment. Studies have shown that ETS is both a safe and effective treatment for PH with success rates over 90%. [6,7] The emergence of uniport surgery and natural orifice transluminal surgery has the potential to further reduce surgical access trauma with promising results. However, controversies still exist concerning the technique and complications relating to ETS, notably the method of sympathetic trunk interruption, the level of interruption and ways to prevent the equally disturbing complication of compensatory hyperhidrosis (CH).

VATS Sympathectomy

Video assisted thoracoscopic surgery (VATS) is widely performed in advanced thoracic centers throughout the world. It is associated with reduced post-operative pain, shorter hospital stay, earlier return to work and fewer overall complications. VATS now plays a major role in the treatment of a wide range of thoracic surgical conditions including major lung resections.

VATS sympathectomy is indicated for patients with severe primary hyperhidrosis suffering from intolerable sweating that persistently interferes with their daily lives. It is important to rule out secondary causes of hyperhidrosis as sympathectomy is not indicated in patients with secondary hyperhidrosis caused by underlying metabolic, infectious or malignant causes. Generally, VATS sympathectomy is the approach of choice when other non-surgical therapies have failed, and for those sufferers seeking a more permanent solution for PH. Success rates have been quoted from 92 to 100%, with particularly promising results in patients with palmar hyperhidrosis. [8]

The principle of sympathectomy is to denervate the eccrine glands by interrupting nerve conduction in the sympathetic chain. Techniques and approaches vary. Methods of interruption of sympathetic chain also range from cauterization, cutting, clipping to division. Some centers advocate ganglionectomy and ramicotomy; while others prefer selective sympathicotomy sparing the ganglions. Sympathicotomy as oppose to more radical denervation procedures usually result in less CH. The level of interruption of the chain is a decision that should be based on the pattern of hyperhidrosis and patient's preference. In an expert consensus, a set of terminology regarding level of interruption has been proposed for better consistency in research and communication. Level of sympathectomy is presented in relation to the rib number. Hence R2 being above the 2nd rib, R3 above the third rib and so on. [9] R3 and R4 interruption yields the driest hands in patients with palmar hyperhidrosis alone, but entails a higher risk of CH. R3 interruption alone may lead to moister hands but lower incidence of CH. Hence, in general, R3 interruption is recommended for patients with palmar hyperhidrosis alone. For craniofacial hyperhidrosis, Chou and colleagues reported CH rate of 27% following R3 only interruption when compared with CH rate of more than 40% following R2 interruption. [10] In another series, R2 and R3 interruption was found to have higher CH rate than R2 alone. [11] Therefore based on these findings, experts suggest R3 only interruption for craniofacial hyperhidrosis for its lower risk of CH.

The conventional bilateral ETS is done with 2 to 3 ports on each side. 10mm ports and 5mm ports are created for the insertion of the camera and dissecting instruments respectively. ETS is done under general anesthesia with double lumen tube intubation and single lung ventilation. An alternative technique for selective upper lobar collapse for sympathectomy has also been described. [12] Depending on surgeon preference, patients are either placed in 30 degrees reversed trendelenburg position with arms abducted or lateral decubitus position. (Figure 1) The former approach allows bilateral ETS to be performed without the need to reposition the patient halfway through the procedure. Bilateral ETS are usually performed in the same session, and patients are discharged later on the same day or day after.

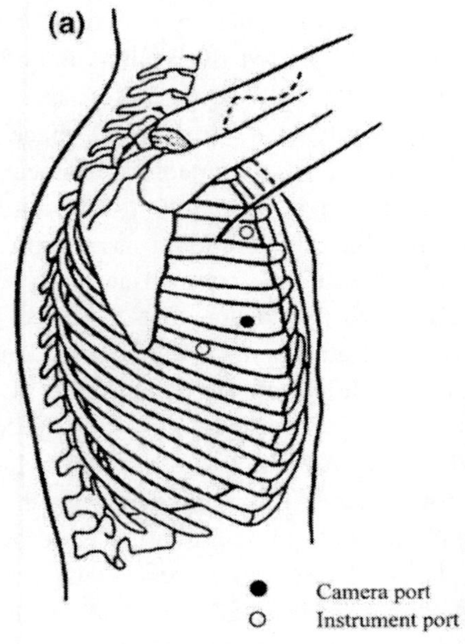

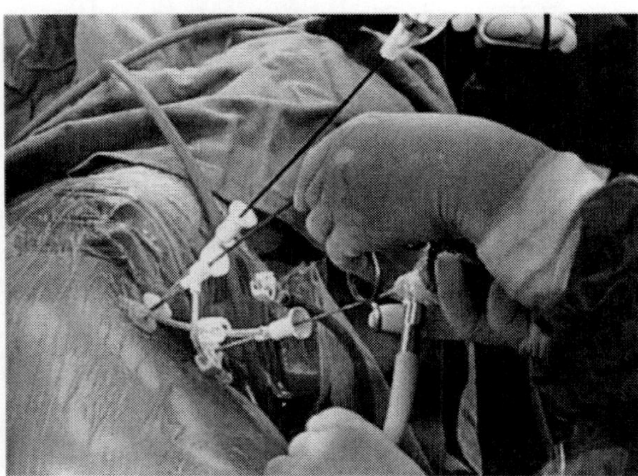

Figure 1. (a) Illustration of a 3-port VATS sympathectomy port placement strategy with patient in lateral decubitus position, (b) Intraoperative photo of 3-port VATS needlescopic sympathectomy.

The introduction of needlescopic instruments allows for even smaller incisions. Technical details of port placement and 2-port or 3-port approaches vary depending on patient anatomy and surgeon preference. The 2-port approach is more commonly used. One such port strategy for the 2-port approach is the insertion of 2mm camera port over 4th or 5th anterior axillary line with the instrument port inserted over midaxillary line in the 3rd or 4th intercostal space. Alternatively, for 3-port needlescopic approach, instrument ports can be inserted anteriorly in 4th intercostal space lateral to pectoralis major muscle ,and posteriorly in 4th intercostal space along the posterior axillary line, with camera port at around 6th -7th intercostal space on mid axillary line. Success rates have been quoted in multiple studies to be above 90%, with complications, excluding compensatory hyperhidrosis, at 5.7 to 9.7%, and 1.9 to 2.7% requiring further post-operative intervention such as chest drain insertion or re- exploration. [6,13] Serious complications that have been reported include pneumothorax (1%), hemothorax (1%) , chylothorax (1%), bradycardia and Horner's syndrome (0.7 – 3%) secondary to damage to stellate ganglion. [9] Rarely, permanent bradycardia has been reported in patients post sympathectomy. The guidelines therefore discourages sympathectomy for patients with preoperative baseline pulse rate of less than 55 per minute. [9] Cases of pacemaker dependent bradycardia have been reported and patients should be warned of risk of reduced exercise capacity post operation. [14] The reported rate of compensatory hyperhidrosis varies in the range of 2.5% to as high as 97% and is the single most significant complication that affects patient satisfaction. In our center's experience, clinical outcomes after needlescopic thoracic sympathectomy by either cauterization or nerve excision for patients with palmar and axillary hyperhidrosis were excellent. At 16-month follow up, there was no recurrence of hyperhidrosis, and 5% developed CH that did not warrant further intervention. [15]

Despite the ultra-minimal invasive nature of needlescopic VATS, chronic postoperative wound sequelaeover thoracic incisions were reported to affect 31.4% of patients in a series. [16] In another study, residual wound pain, numbness and paresthesia were also reported in around 40% of patients. [17] Over 15% of patients also experienced residual shoulder joint dysfunction and paresthesia over wound in post needlescopic surgery. In our series, the rate of paresthesia was 50% post needlescopic sympathectomy, with 17.6 % of patients experiencing the symptom 12 months post-surgery. However, the paresthesia did not seem to affect patient satisfaction from the sympathectomy procedure. [18]

The debate on whether cauterizing, clipping or ablation of the sympathetic chain achieves better symptom resolution is ongoing, and so far no discernible difference among different techniques has been reported, provided the sympathectomy is done properly with enough separation between ends of chain to prevent regrowth. [19] The proposed extent of lateral cauterization of communicating fibres (Fibres of Kuntz) is around 2-3 cm lateral to the sympathetic ganglion.

Uniportal (Single Port) Endoscopic Sympathectomy

Uniportal endoscopic surgery is a maturing technique in thoracic surgery. One stage bilateral uniportal sympathectomy can be safely and successfully performed, and is increasingly practiced around the world. Studies have shown uniportal surgery has benefits over conventional ETS in terms of less post-operative pain, better aesthetics and shorter operative time. [20,21] Furthermore, the efficacy and rates of compensatory hyperhidrosis are not inferior to conventional ETS.

Many different methods of uniportal surgery have been reported. [22,23] The majority of cases are done under general anesthesia with double lumen intubation and single- lung ventilation. Patients can be positioned in the semi-sitting position with 90 degrees abduction of the upper limbs or the lateral decubitus position. Usually, a single incision is made over the anterior axillary line around 3rd to 4th intercostal space lateral to the pectoralis major muscle bilaterally, and the length of the incision is around 8mm to 1 cm. Various instruments have been reportedly used for uniportal sympathectomy, and the number of instrument inserted into the incision also varies. The initial report utilized a modified pediatric urology cystoureteroscopy for the bilateral procedure. [22] Subsequently, Rocco described the technique of using more conventional endoscopic instruments such as the 3mm thoracoscope and 5mm endoscopic dissector to accomplish the sympathectomy. However, this requires insertion of two instruments into a small incision which may result in fencing and undesirable movements of the endoscope. Recently, the use of Vasoview Hemopro 2 dissector for sympathectomy was reported. (Figure 2) Originally designed for endoscopic vein harvesting, the multifunctional single instrument module allows uniportal sympathectomy without the need to fit multiple instruments into one small incision. [24] The instrument consists of a

7mm high resolution endoscope, a parallel working channel for the Hemopro 2 dissector, a built in CO2 gas insufflation channel and retractable lens cleaning system all incorporated into the 12 mm diameter Vasoview device. The design of the Hemopro 2 grasper and scissors contain unique thermostatic designs which can reduce collateral thermal tissue damage during cutting and cauterization. So far no direct comparisons have been made between different uniport techniques.

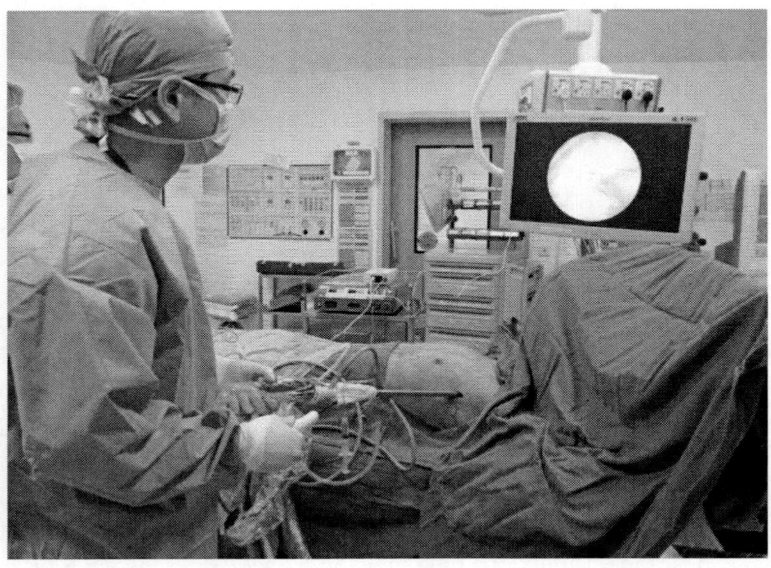

Figure 2. Operating room set up, position, and access for bilateral uniportal Vasoview® sympathectomy.

Results of uniportal surgery have been encouraging. In a series of 130 patients undergoing uniport ETS for palmar hyperhidrosis, there was 100% symptom resolution, with reported quality of life improvement in over 90%. The rate of CH was 19%, and none of the patients experienced residual pain during follow-up on postoperative day 7. The major complication rate was 0.35%. Mean operation time was 38 minutes with mean hospital stay of 1.1 days. [25] Another study reported 97% of patients with 2 point reduction in the hyperhidrosis severity score after receiving uniport ETS of mixed methods and approach with Vasoview or paediatric GAAB neuroendoscopes. Out of the 100 patients, only 13% required analgesics during the first week following their surgery. [26] In our center, 16 patients underwent Vasoview bilateral VATS sympathectomy for severe palmar hyperhidrosis. All procedures were successful with resolution of hyperhidrosis in all patients. Mean operative time was 56 minutes for bilateral procedures, and there was no conversion to larger incisions. Mean post-operative stay was < 1 day and the post operation VAS pain score at discharge was 1.8. [27] In a study comparing uniportal ETS and 2-port ETS, Chen et al. found uniportal ETS to be equally safe and effective as conventional ETS, with less postoperative pain and shorter operative time. (39.5 vs 49.7 minutes). [20] While more stringent studies are needed to substantiate the benefit of uniportal ETS over conventional ETS, with the maturation of the uniport technique, surgeons are increasingly comfortable in practicing uniport surgery. Patients should be adequately consented to be able to choose between conventional ETS and uniport ETS depending on available expertise. [28]

Embryonic Natural Orifice Endoscopic Surgery

The development of embryonic natural orifice endoscopic surgery (ENOTES) has garnered interest among surgeons recently for the treatment of hyperhidrosis. The rationale behind the development of ENOTES is to avoid thoracic incisions that may be unsightly, and the potential chronic pain and discomfort associated with surgical access through the thoracic cage.

Zhu et al. reported a novel technique for ENOTES sympathectomy with access via the umbilicus. After placing the patient under general anesthesia and double lumen intubation, a 5mm incision was made over the umbilicus. Pneumoperitoneum was achieved at 10mmHg CO2 under the guidance of an ultrathin gastroscope and the thoracic cavity was entered via the muscular portions of the diaphragm with a 5mm needle knife. T3 ganglionectomy was performed with a hot biopsy forceps for patients with palmar hyperhidrosis; and T3 + T4 ganglionectomy performed for patients with palmar and axillary hyperhidrosis. Accessory fibres and nerves of Kuntz were then cauterized up to 2 cm lateral to the ganglion. In their series of 35 patients successfully treated for palmar hyperhidrosis, the average hospital stay was 1 day and the mean operation time was 65 minutes. No major complications were reported. The rate of compensatory hyperhidrosis was around 28.6% in 1 year. Overall 88.5% of the patients reported improvement in quality of life and over 75% were very satisfied with the surgery. At 14 months follow-up, 97% of the patients remained symptom free, and almost all the patients were satisfied with the cosmetic results of the surgery. [29] In a comparative study between ENOTES and needlescopic sympathectomy, ENOTES was found to be comparable with VATS sympathectomy in terms of efficacy and complications. Despite the longer operative time (56 vs 40 minutes), patients underwent ENOTES had reduced post-operative pain and paresthesia at all-time intervals. There was no report of intra-abdominal complications at 1.4 years follow-up. [30]

The true value of ENOTES and its added benefit over conventional or uniport ETS remains to be investigated. Larger studies with longer follow-up are needed to address issues such as added risk of intrabdominal complications so as to allow surgeons and patients a more accurate measurement of ENOTES's overall value. Nonetheless, ENOTES may represent an alternative for patients who do not wish to have thoracic incisions or have had previous surgery around the chest.

Robotic Sympathectomy

Some studies have suggested that lower rates of compensatory hyperhidrosis are associated with selective post ganglionic ramicotomy compared to ganglionectomy. [31] [32] However, technically, selective ramicotomies is challenging with conventional ETS due to restricted maneuverability and 2 dimensional visualization of the anatomy. Coveliers et al. reported a novel technique of robotic ETS to perform selective postganglionic ramicotomies for 55 patients. [33] The advantage of robotic ETS to conventional ETS is that it can provide the surgeon with better 3 dimensional visualization and instrument maneuverability in a confined space, facilitating selective ramicotomies. With the patient in the lateral decubitus position, three 2 cm incisions were made at the tip of scapula and the costal arch, with an additional incision for camera. The right and left robotic arms, along with the hook cautery were introduced into the thoracic cavity after one lung ventilation. Ribs 2, 3 and 4 were pre-marked, and division of rami from T2 to T4, nerves of Kuntz and accessary fibres was performed, with margins up to 2cm lateral to the sympathetic chain. Postoperative drains were placed and subsequently removed once the patient was out of surgery. Of the 110 sympathectomies performed, the resolution rate of PH was 96% after 24 months follow up. The rate of compensatory hyperhidrosis was 7.2%. The median hospital stay was 1 day and the median operative time was 80 minutes.

Interestingly, another study randomized VATS sympathectomy procedures to compare robotic versus human camera holding. The results showed that camera holding by robotic arm was equally safe and effective as human camera holding VATS, but was less efficient and required a longer surgery time. There was no discernible difference in rates of CH between the 2 groups. [34] Therefore, it remains uncertain whether robotic sympathectomy is a worthwhile alternative for treatment of PH in the absence of meaningful cost analysis and significant benefits. In addition, the creation of multiple incisions during robotic sympathectomy may create more wound related complications. The overall efficacy and beneficial effect of robotic ETS remains to be further rigorously validated.

Compensatory Hyperhidrosis

Compensatory hyperhidrosis is a significant complication of sympathectomy. It is the major reason behind poor quality of life and dissatisfaction following sympathectomy, and may even lead to patient regret over the procedure. CH most commonly occurs over the back, followed by the chest, abdomen and face. It is hypothesized to be related to extensive dissection and ganglionectomy, with resulting disruption of communication within the sympathetic chain. Higher sympathetic blockade disrupts larger number of afferent inhibitory fibres that dampen sudomotor output from the hypothalamus leading to hyperhidrosis. CH, similar to primary hyperhidrosis is also found to be driven by external stressors or exercise which lends weight to the hypothesis that CH maybe a physiological response for thermoregulation after the total surface area for body cooling and sweating is reduced with successful denervation after sympathectomy. Studies to find methods to reduce the incidence of CH have drawn variable recommendations because of heterogeneity among techniques, assessment methods and studied population. The rate of CH varies with studies, ranging from 3- 98%. The lowest reported rate of CH is 2.5% in a series of patients with transthoracic selective sympathectomy performed on post ganglionic fibers emanating from the 2nd to 4th sympathetic ganglia, while most studies report incidence around 50 to 80%. The rate of severe CH significantly affecting quality of life and producing persistent staining of clothes is around 12-15%. Rodriguez et al. reported 6% of patients regretting surgery due to compensatory hyperhidrosis. [35] While the occurrence of CH is unpredictable, some studies report a correlation between lower level sympathectomy with lower incidence and severity of CH. Apparently being female is also a predictor of suffering from CH. Selective ramicotomy without damage to the ganglion is also reported to have a lower incidence of CH. In an expert consensus, T2 ganglion interruption is a risk factor for CH. For palmar hyperhidrosis alone, R3 and R4 interruption has a higher risk of CH, but yields the best dry hands, while R4 interruption alone has lower incidence of CH, but may result in moister hands. [9, 36,37] Other techniques have been described to minimize the degree of CH. Interruption of the sympathetic chain by applying surgical clips onto the nerve has been reported in small studies, and this method is favoured by some surgeons as it is potentially reversible. The rationale behind is that if patients develop CH postoperatively, "unclipping" of the chain can be done to improve or ameliorate symptoms. However, this method of clipping remains less popular because of possible higher incidence of "sympathectomy" failure, and the unproven value of unclipping in managing severe CH. The clipping technique is still considered by experts to be irreversible.

The symptoms of severe CH can be extremely debilitating, and reconnection of the sympathetic chain, for example by nerve graft, may have a role in improving symptoms. Hamm et al. reported their case series on VATS reversal of sympathectomy in 19 patients by using an intercostal nerve graft. The process involved anastomosing the somatic nerve graft with an autonomic efferent nerve to restore the somatic- central nervous system reflex arc. In that series, 9 (47%) patients experienced significant improvement in their compensatory hyperhidrosis. [38] In our center, the needlescopic VATS approach for sympathectomy reversal has been performed on a patient suffering from debilitating CH and post sympathectomy heatstroke. A segment of the fourth intercostal nerve was harvested as a free graft and joined to the free ends of the sympathetic chain with fibrin sealant. The patient reported improvements in subjective compensatory sweating and also noted reappearance of palmar sweating but not to the extent of hyperhidrosis. He was able to resume work following surgery, and could reengage in physical exercise without further problems. [39] The exact clinical and physiological implication of this treatment is still under investigation. However it may provide a viable option for patients who wish to achieve amelioration of CH surgically. The use of medications such as oxybutynin and Botox are also options to treating CH. The details of these therapies and medications are beyond the scope of this article.

Conclusion

Endoscopic thoracic sympathectomy is the treatment of choice for patients with primary hyperhidrosis as it provides lasting symptomatic relief. Despite the complication of compensatory hyperhidrosis, the majority of patients is highly satisfied with the post operation results and enjoys a better quality of life. With the advent and emergence of uniport ETS and ENOTES, access trauma may be further reduced without compromising the overall efficacy of the surgery. To date, no definite technique is proven to be the "ideal surgery", as each method has its merits and shortcomings. Interestingly, the different methods and approaches for sympathectomy do not seem to significantly alter symptom resolution, patient satisfaction and rates of complication. Compensatory hyperhidrosis remains a challenging clinical problem in post sympathectomy patients. This makes pre-operative assessment and communication with patients of paramount importance. Patients should be counseled sufficiently on the success rates of surgery and the potential complications associated. Patient's tolerance of residual and compensatory hyperhidrosis should be explored adequately before any decision is reached as there is no effective remedy for severe compensatory hyperhidrosis to date. The introduction of newer techniques for more selective sympathectomy by utilizing the robot, and for treatment of CH by reestablishing sympathetic nerve integrity, such as intercostal nerve grafting, may provide answers to ameliorate this disturbing complication. Ultimately, the introduction of minimally invasive thoracic sympathectomy, along with its evolving techniques, should improve the quality of life of patients with a debilitating condition such as primary hyperhidrosis.

References

[1] Strutton DR, Kowalski J, Glaser DA, Stang PE. US prevalence of hyperhidrosis and impact on individuals with axillary hyperhidrosis: results from a national survey. *J. Am. Acad. Dermatol.* 2004; 51: 241-248.

[2] Leung AK, Chan PY, Choi MC. Hyperhidrosis. *Int. J. Dermatol.* 1999;28:561-7.

[3] Epidemiological survey of primary palmar hyperhidrosis in adolescent in Fuzhou of People's Republic of China. *Eur. J. Cardiothorac. Surg.* 2007; 31:737-9.

[4] Kotzareff A. Resection partielle de trone sympathetique cervical droit pour hyperhidrosis unilateral. *Rev. Med. Suisse Romande* 1920;40:111-3.

[5] Kux F. The endoscopic approach to the vegetative nervous system and its therapeutic possibilities: especially in duodenal ulcer, angina pectoris, hypertension , diabetes. *Dis. Chest.* 1951;20(2) : 139 – 147.

[6] Askari A, Kordzadeh A, Lee GH, Harvey M. Endoscopic thoracic sympathectomy for primary hyperhidrosis: 16-year follow up in a single UK centre. *Surgeon* 2013; 11:130-3.

[7] Atkinson LD, Forde-Thomas NC, Fealey RD Endoscopic Transthoracic Limited Sympathotomy for Palmar – Plantar Hyperhidrosis : Outcomes and Complications During a 10-year period. *Mayo Clin. Proc.* 2011:869:721-729.

[8] Bell D, Jedynak D, Bell R. Predictors of outcome following endoscopic thoracic sympathectomy. *ANZ J. Surg.* 2014;84(1-2):68-72.

[9] Cerfolio RJ, De Campos JR, Bryant AS, Connery CP, Millar DL, DeCamp MM, et al. The Society of Thoracic Surgery expert consensus for the surgical treatment of hyperhidrosis. *Ann. Thorac. Surg.* 2011;91:1642–8.

[10] Chou SH , Kao EL , Lin CC, Chang YT, Huang MF. The importance of classification in sympathetic surgery and a proposed mechanism for compensatory hyperhidrosis : experience with 464 cases. *Surg. Endosc.* 2006 ; 20:1749-53.

[11] Licht PB, Ladegaard L, Pilegaard HK. Thoracoscopic sympathectomy for isolated facial blushing. *Ann. Thorac. Surg* 2006 ;11:59-62.

[12] Sihoe AD, Ho KM, Sze TS, Lee TW, Yim AP. Selective lobar collapse for video-assisted thoracic surgery. *Ann. Thorac. Surg.* 2004;77(1):278-83.

[13] Plas EG , Fugger R, Herbst F, Fritsch A. Complications of endoscopic thoracic sympathectomy. *Surgery* 1995;118:493-5.

[14] Lai CL, Chen WJ, Liu YB, Lee YT. Bradycardia and permanent pacing after bilateral thoracoscopic T2 sympathectomy for primary hyperhidrosis. *Pacing Clin. Electrophysiol.* 2001; 24:524-5.

[15] Yim APC, Liu HP, Lee TW, Wan S, Arifi AA. 'Needlescopic' video-assisted thoracic surgery for palmar hyperhidrosis. *Eur. J. Cardiothorac. Surg* 2000; 17: 697–701.

[16] Hutter J, Miller K, Moritz E. Chronic sequels after thoracoscopic procedures for benign diseases. *Eur. J. Cardiothorac. Surg.* 2000;17: 687-690.

[17] Steegers MA, Snik DM, Verhagen AF, van der Drift MS, Wilder Smith OH. Only half of chronic pain after thoracic surgery shows a neuropathic component. *J. Pain.* 2008;9:955-61.

[18] Sihoe AD, Cheung CS, Lai HK, Lee TW, Thung KH, Yim AP. Incidence of chest wall paresthesia after needlescopic video-assisted thoracic surgery for palmar hyperhidrosis. *Eur. J. Cardiothorac. Surg.* 2005;27:313–9.

[19] Yanagihara TK , Ibrahimiye A, Harris C et al. Analysis of clamping versus cutting of T3 sympathetic nerve for severe palmar hyperhidrosis. *J. Thorac. Cardiovasc. Surg* 2010 ; 140 : 984-9.

[20] Chen YB, Ye W, Yang WT et al. Uniportal versus biportal video-assisted thoracoscopic sympathectomy for palmar hyperhidrosis. *Chinese Medical Journal*, vol. 122, no. 13, pp 1525-1528.

[21] Lin TS, Kuo SJ, Chou MC. Uniportal endoscopic thoracic sympathectomy for treatment of palmar and axillary hyperhidrosis; analysis of 2000 cases. *Neurosurgery* 2002;51 (suppl) : S84 – S87.

[22] Lardinois D, Ris HB. Minimally invasive video-endoscopic sympathectomy by use of a transaxillary single port approach. *Eur. J. Cardiothorac Surg* 2002; 21: 67–70.

[23] Rocco G. Endoscopic VATS sympathectomy: the uniportal technique. Multimed Man Cardiothorac Surg. 2007 Jan 1;2007(507):MMCTS. 2004.000323doi: 10.1510/MMCTS.2004.000323.

[24] Ng CSH, Yeung ECL, Wong RHL, Kwok WT. Single-port Sympathectomy for Palmar Hyperhidrosis with VasoView HemoPro 2 Endoscopic Vein Harvesting Device. *J. Thorac. Cardiovasc. Surg.* 2012 Nov;144(5):1256-7.

[25] Mohsen Ibrahim, Cecilia Menna, Claudio Andreettti et al. Clinical study.Bilateral single port sympathectomy: Long term results and quality of life. *BioMed Research International* 2013 October article ID 348017.

[26] Kujipers M, Theo J Klinkenberg, Wobbe Bouma, Mike J DeJongtse , Massimo A Mariani. Single port one-stage bilateral thoracoscopic sympathicotomy for severe hyperhidrosis: prospective analysis of a standardized approach. *Journal of Cardiothoracic Surgery* 2013, 8 : 216.

[27] Ng CSH, Lau RWH, Wong RHL, Ho AMH, Wan S. Single Port Vasoview Sympathectomy for Palmar Hyperhidrosis: A Clinical Update.

Journal of Laparoendoscopic & Advanced Surgical Techniques 2014;24(1):32-4.

[28] Ng CSH, Lau RWH, Wong RHL, Yim APC. Evolving Techniques of Endoscopic Thoracic Sympathectomy: Smaller Incisions or Less? *The Surgeon* 2013;11:290-291.

[29] Zhu LH, Du Q, Chen L, Yang S, Tu Y, Chen S, Chen W. One-year follow-up period after transumbilical thoracic sympathectomy for hyperhidrosis: outcomes and consequences. *J. Thorac. Cardiovasc. Surg.* 2014 Jan;147(1):25-8.

[30] Zhu LH, Chen L, Yang S, Liu D, Zhang J, Cheng X, Chen W. Embryonic NOTES thoracic sympathectomy for palmar hyperhidrosis: results of a novel technique and comparison with the conventional VATS procedure. *Surg Endosc.* 2013 Nov;27(11):4124-9 [

[31] Lee DY, Paik HC, Kim DH, Kim HW. Comparative analysis of T3 selective division of rami communicantes (ramicotomy) to T3 sympathetic clipping in treatment of palmar hyperhidrosis. *Clin. Auton. Res.* 2003;13 Suppl 1:I45-7.

[32] Friedel g, Linder A, Toomes H. Sympathectomy and vagotomy. In: Mannecke K, Rosin RD , eds. Minimal access thoracic surgery. First edition. Philadelphia : Lippimcott- Raven publishing 1998 : 67 -83.

[33] Coveliers H, Meyer M, Gharagozloo F, Wisselink W, Rauwerda J, Margolis M, Tempesta B, Strother E. Robotic selective postganglionic thoracic sympathectomy for the treatment of hyperhidrosis. *Ann. Thorac. Surg.* 2013 Jan;95(1):269-74.

[34] Martins Rua JF, Jatene FB, de Campos JR, Monteiro R, Tedde ML, Samano MN, Bernardo WM, Das-Neves-Pereira JC. Robotic versus human camera holding in video-assisted thoracic sympathectomy: a single blind randomized trial of efficacy and safety. *Interact. Cardiovasc. Thorac. Surg.* 2009 Feb;8(2):195.

[35] Rodríguez PM, Freixinet JL, Hussein M, Valencia JM, Gil RM, Herrero J, et al. Side effects, complications and outcome of thoracoscopic sympathectomy for palmar and axillary hyperhidrosis in 406 patients. *Eur. J. Cardiothorac. Surg.* 2008;34:514–9.

[36] Liu Y, Yang J. Liu J et al. Surgical treatment of primary palmar hyperhidrosis: a prospective randomized study comparing T3- T4 sympathicotomy. *Eur. J. Cardiothorac. Surg.* 2009 ;35:398-402.

[37] Yang J , Tan JJ, Ye GL,Gu WQ, Wang J, liu YG. T3/T4 thoracic sympathicotomy and compensatory sweating in treatment of palmar hyperhidrosis. *Chin. Med. J.* 2007;120:1574-7.

[38] Haam SJ, Park SY, Paik HC, Lee DY. Sympathetic nerve reconstruction for compensatory hyperhidrosis after sympathetic surgery for primary hyperhidrosis. *J. Korean Med. Sci.* 2010;25:597–601.

[39] Wong RHL, Ng CSH, Wong JKW, Tsang S. Needlescopic video-assisted thoracic surgery for reversal of thoracic sympathectomy. *Interact. CardioVasc. Thorac. Surg.* 2012;14:350-2.

In: Hyperhidrosis
Editor: Janine R. Huddle

ISBN: 978-1-63321-516-0

Chapter IV

Hyperhidrosis: A Brief Overview

Eshini Perera [1,2] ***and Rodney Sinclair*** [1,2]
[1]The University of Melbourne, Melbourne, Victoria, Australia
[2]Sinclair Dermatology, Melbourne, Victoria Australia

Abstract

Hyperhidrosis is a common condition which is troublesome for patients and carries a significant psychosocial burden. Hyperhidrosis can be either generalised of focal. Treatment may require oral anticholinergic agents. Focal hyperhidrosis is usually primary and responds to topical measures. Specialist referral for botulinum toxin A, iontophoresis or sympathectomy should be considered for severe cases. This article details an approach to the assessment and managment of hyperhidrosis and outlines the current treatment options that are available.

Introduction

Hyperhidrosis is a disorder characterized by the increased production of sweat disproportionate to the amount required to compensate for environmental conditions or thermoregulatory needs. [1]

It is estimated to affect about 3% of the general population, [2] affecting both men and woman equally. The pathophysiology of hyperhidrosis is poorly understood, however, dysfunction of the sympathetic nervous system, particularly the cholinergic fibres that innervate the eccrine glands, is postulated [1]

This condition can be deeply distressing for patients causing both physical discomfort and social awkwardness however a recent survey demonstrates that only one third of participants seek input from their general practitioners. [2] Hyperhidrosis may impact daily activities of living and impair performance and productivity of work.

Patients also experience higher rates of depression and reduced levels of confidence. [2]

Sensitive management of hyperhidrosis by general practitioners can help reduce the psychosocial impact.

Table 1. Causes of generalised hyperhidrosis

Endocrine diseases:
  - Diabetes **
  - Hyperthyroidism *
  - Pheochromocytoma ***
  - Hyperpituitarism ***
  - Hypoglycaemia **
  - Menopause *
  - Carcinoid syndrome ***
- Malignancy ***
- Febrile infective illness **
  - Malaria **
  - Tuberculosis **
  - Endocarditis **
- Congestive heart failure **
- Neurological disorders **
  - Parkinson's disease **
  - Peripheral neuropathies **
  - Brain lesions e.g malformation of corpus callosum **
- Drugs *

* uncommon
** very uncommon
*** rare

Assessment and Diagnosis of Hyperhidrosis

Hyperhidrosis can be generalized or focal. Generalized hyperhidrosis affects the entire body and may be idiopathic or secondary to an underlying metabolic disorder or systemic disease. A number of conditions that have been associated with generalised hyperhidrosis are listed in Table 1.

Most of these conditions can be identified on history and examination. Patients most likely to require further investigation are those who are older, or those with severe hyperhidrosis of recent onset. Investigations that may be helpful are listed in Table 2.

Table 2. Investigations that may be considered for last onset, recent onset or very severe hyperhidrosis

- FBC
- UEC
- LFT
- TFT
- Fasting glucose level
- HIV
- Testing for various infective disease including TB, malaria etc if patient's history is suggestive of exposure.
- 24 hour urinary catecholamines

Table 3. Causes of focal hyperhidrosis

- Primary idiopathic hyperhidrosis
- Gustatory sweating (sweating after eating or seeing food which produces strong salivation. Chewing can also stimulate sweating)
- Neurological causes
  - Spinal injuries
  - Neuropathies

Focal hyperhidrosis involves specific sites of the body, most commonly the axilla, palms and soles. Focal hyperhidrosis occurs in otherwise healthy patients commonly before the age of 25 years [3], and roughly two-thirds of patients report a positive family history. [1] The most common cause of focal hyperhidrosis is primary idiopathic hyperhidrosis however other causes are outlined in Table 3. It is important to note that primary hyperhidrosis ceases when sleeping, in contrast to night sweats, which can indicate a serious underlying disorder. A distinction between generalized and focal hyperhidrosis should be made at the initial assessment. The medical history should be concentrated on:

- location of sweating: general or specific area, unilateral or symmetrical areas
- duration of presentation
- family history of focal hyperhidrosis
- age of onset
- concurrent medical illnesses
- triggers of sweating including anxiety, chewing, eating, temperature.

A diagnosis of idiopathic focal hyperhidrosis can be made on history if the patient is noted to have excessive visible sweating for at least 6 months and two of the following:

- bilateral symmetrical sweating
- impairment of daily activities
- at least one episode per week
- onset before 25 years of age
- positive family history
- focal sweating that ceases during sleep.

If there is no obvious underlying cause on history and examination, and the presentation is characteristic for primary focal hyperhidrosis, then further investigations are not required.

An Overview of the Management of Hyperhydrosis

There are a number of treatments available both surgically and non-surgically for the treatment of focal hyperhidrosis. Management of generalised hyperhidrosis, on the other hand, involves addressing the underlying cause.

Topical Therapies for Focal Hyperhidrosis

Aluminium Compounds

While most standard supermarket antiperspirants contain aluminium chloride, higher potency agents may contain aluminium chlorohydrate. Aluminium chloride hexhydrate is significantly more effective again, and should be the first line of therapy. Antiperspirants containing aluminium chloride hexhydrate are sold in pharmacies; a prescription is not required.

All of these agents have a common mechanism of action that involves the mechanical obstruction of the eccrine gland duct, which in turn leads to atrophy of the eccrine acini. [4]

Aluminium chloride hexhydrate is used in a concentration of 20% for axillary hyperhidrosis, while 25% for palmar and plantar hyperhidrosis is usually needed to achieve euhydrosis. [5, 6] However, a concentration of 10% can be used initially to avoid side effects, including localised skin irritation and a burning sensation.

Topical therapy should be applied once daily, usually at night when the skin is dry, for optimal results. The concentration can be increased up to 35%, as tolerated, if there is no response, although patients can rarely tolerate side effects at this strength in the axilla. Associated skin irritation can be controlled with 1% hydrocortisone. Aluminium chloride hexhydrate in higher strengths may be tolerated on the palms and soles and can be mixed with salicylic acid gel or ethanol to maximise effectiveness in these areas.

Iontophoresis

Iontophoresis is a specialised treatment only available in some states. It utilises a delivery system for small polar molecules into the skin (Figure 1). Figure 2 and Figure 3 provide a visual comparison for the effectiveness of this therapy. The most effective chemical for hyperhidrosis is glycopyrrolate. The effectiveness of glycopyrrolate over tap water has been documented a number of times within the literature. [7, 8, 9] While tap water is much less effective, there are iontophoresis devices available for home use. [10]

Botulinum Toxin A

Botulinum toxin A is a highly effective treatment for focal hyperhidrosis. The main mechanism of action is the inhibition of acetylcholine release from the sympathetic nerves that innervate the eccrine sweat glands.[11] The dose for intradermal injections depend on the area, eg. 50–100 U for the axilla. The treatment is highly effective for palmar and planter hyperhidrosis, although pain during injections can be a limiting factor to its use.

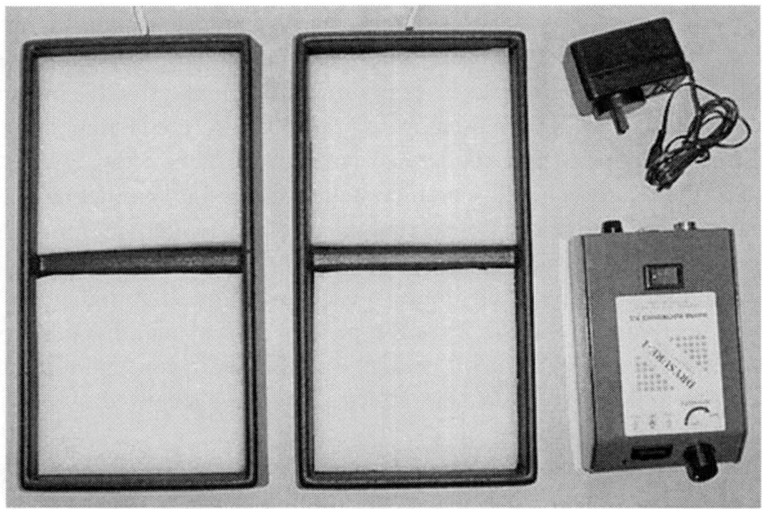

Figure 1. An iontophoresis machine.

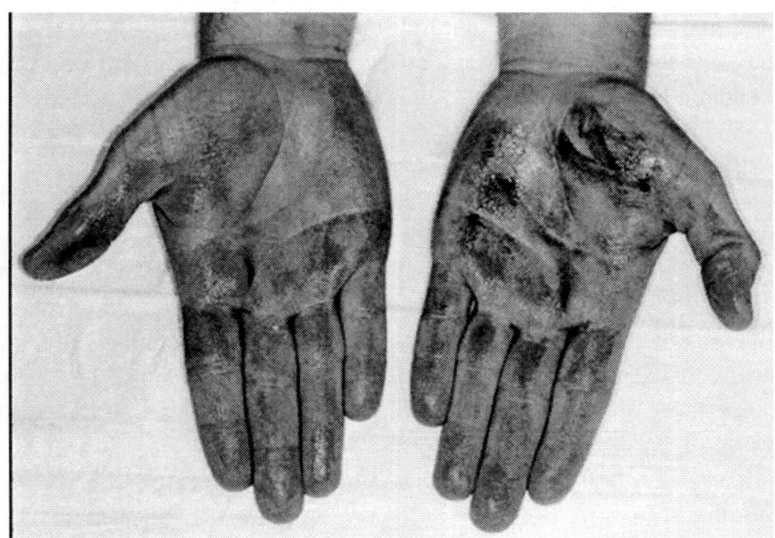

Figure 2. The starch-iodine test. Iodine is applied to a dry area of skin and starch is sprinkled on top. The iodine, starch and sweat react to form the dark sediment. The left palm has not yet been treated with iontophoresi.

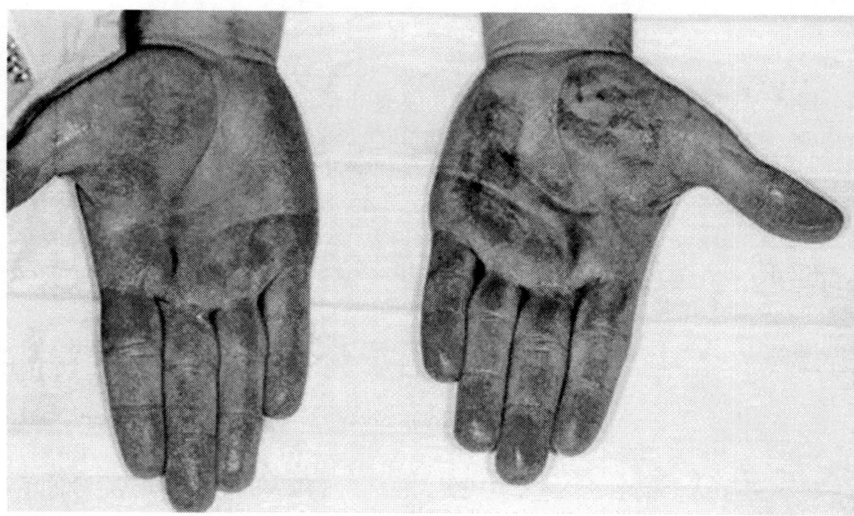

Figure 3. Starch-iodine test after a patient has had iontophoresis to the left palm 7 days earlier. The image demonstrates a reduction in perspiration.

Systemic Therapy

There is long term data on the safety and efficacy of anticholinergic use in focal hyperhidrosis. Propantheline bromide and oxybutynin are the most common anticholinergics used. Both are highly effective and relatively cheap. Selective serotonin reuptake inhibitor (SSRI) induced hyperhidrosis also responds well to oxybutynin. Glycopyrrolate is another effective alternative, but expense is a limiting factor for many patients.The dosage required to control hyperhidrosis invariably results in generalised anticholinergic effects, including dry mouth and eyes, urinary retention and headaches.

Oxybutynin can be prescribed initially at a low dose of 2.5 mg/day and increased progressively up to 10 mg/day until an improvement is seen. This regimen results in fewer side effects. [12]

The Role of Surgery

Surgery is reserved for those refractory to medical therapy and in whom the hyperhidrosis is having a significant impact on their activities of daily living. Local excision of the axillary vault may reduce excessive sweating in the axilla. The results, however, can be cosmetically unappealing and scarring can result in functional impairment. Removal of axillary sweat glands using tumescent liposuction has also been shown to be a safe method of reducing axillary hyperhidrosis. [13] The cost of this procedure may be a limiting factor for some patients, particularly as there is a risk of relapse of hyperhidrosis. [13]

Endoscopic thoracic sympathectomy is the last resort for the treatment of palmar, axillary and craniofacial hyperhidrosis and works by interrupting the fibers of the sympathetic ganglia. The cost, which starts from $5000, can make this an unacceptable option for many patients. Secondly, the surgery itself has many risks. These risks include Horner's syndrome, pneumothorax and more commonly compensatory hyperhidrosis, the latter occurring in 67% of patients who have had endoscopic thoracic sympathectomy. [14]

Conclusion

Hyperhidrosis is a distressing conditions and greatly impact on quality of life on both a social and functional level. Assessment should discriminate between generalized and focal hyperhidrosis and should also focus on the impact the condition has on the patient's life. Conservative treatment measures should be trialed first prior to referral for more invasive treatment. Even though a significant effect on quality of life has been identified only a handful of patients seek advice from their general practitioner. Early identification can reduce the impact excessive sweating has on activities of daily living and social functioning.

References

[1] Solish N, Bertucci V, Dansereua A, et al. A comprehensive approach to the recognition, diagnosis, and severity-based treatment of focal hyperhidrosis: Recommendations of the Canadian Hyperhidrosis Advisory Committee. *Dermatol. Surg.* 2007;33:908–23.

[2] Strutton D, Kowalsk J, Glaser D, et al. U.S prevalence of hyperhidrosis and impact on individuals with axillary hyperhidrosis: results from a national survey. *J. Am. Acad. Dermatol.* 2004;51:241–8.

[3] Haider A, Solish N. Focal hyperhidrosis: diagnosis and management. *Can. Med. Assoc. J.* 2005;172:69–75.

[4] Holzle E, Braun-Falco O. Structural changes in axillary eccrine glands following long-term treatment with aluminium chloride hexahydrate solution. *Br. J. Dermatol.* 1984;110:399–403.

[5] Scholes K, Crow K, Ellis J, et al. Axillary hyperhidrosis treated with alcoholic solution of aluminium chloride hexahydrate. *BMJ* 1978;2: 84–5.

[6] Walling H, Swick B. Treatment options for hyperhidrosis. *Am. J. Clin.* Dermatol 2011;12:285–95.

[7] Abell E, Morgan K. The treatment of idiopathic hyperhidrosis by glycopyrronium bromide and tap water iontophoresis. *Br. J. Dermatol.* 1974;91:87–91.

[8] Bajaj V, Langtry J. Use of oral glycopyrronium bromide in hyperhidrosis. *Br. J. Dermatol.* 2007;157:118–21.

[9] Askari S, Glaser D, King R, Oliver D. Comparison of tap water iontophoresis to iontophoresis with glycopyrrolate. *J. Am. Acad. Dermatol.* 2008;58(S2):AB32.

[10] Dolianitis C, Scarff C, Kelly J, Sinclair R. Iontophoresis with glycopyrrolate for the treatment of palmoplantar hyperhidrosis. *Aust. J. Dermatol.* 2004;45:208–12.

[11] Connolly M, de Berker D, Management of primary hyperhidrosis. Am. *J. Clin Dermatol.* 2003;4:681–97.

[12] Wolosker N, Milanez de Campos J, Kauffman P, et al. The use of oxybutynin for treating axillary hyperhidrosis. *Ann. Vasc. Surg.* 2011;25:1057–62.

[13] Lee M, Ryman W. Liposuction for axillary hyperhidrosis. *Aust. J. Dermatol.* 2005;46:76–9.

[14] Herbst F, Plas E, Fugger R, et al. Endoscopic thoracic sympathectomy for primary hyperhidrosis of the upper limbs: a critical analysis and long-term results of 480 operations. *Ann. Surg.* 1994;220:86–90.

In: Hyperhidrosis
Editor: Janine R. Huddle
ISBN: 978-1-63321-516-0

Chapter V

Pay for Performance? – Can Quality of Life Be Considered in Decision Making Process of Treatment Choice For Patients with Primary Focal Hyperhidrosis? A Review of Epidemiology, Guidelines, Treatment Options, Quality of Life Instruments and Treatment Costs

Christian Müller[1*]***, Corinna Bachmann***[2]
and Paul Kamudoni[3]
[1]Hausen, Germany
[2]Rheinfelden, Germany
[3]London, England

* Corresponding Author: Dr. Christian Müller, Bergwerkstr. 12a, 79688 Hausen; E-Mail: cjmueller@gmx.de; Tel.: 0049 1515 8741397.

Abstract

Primary focal hyperhidrosis is a common disorder with significant impact on occupational, physical, emotional and social life. A systematic review of current literature for primary focal hyperhidrosis was performed with focus on guidelines, epidemiology and quality of life instruments. The relation between treatment option, quality of life outcome, measured as Hyperhidrosis Disease Severity Scale (HDSS) or Dermatology Life Quality Index (DLQI), and rare treatment costs have been investigated. There are numerous instruments available to measure the quality of life (QOL) of the hyperhidrosis patient. In practice, however, only a few (HDSS, DLQI) are used. Additionally, treatment with Botulinum Toxin A seems to be the cheapest for primary focal hyperhidrosis. No relationship of cost-effectiveness and decision-making process for hyperhidrosis treatment choice could be found. For future decision-making processes the dermatologist remains to evaluate not only the severity of hyperhidrosis to achieve the best therapeutic outcome, but also to measure quality of life in order to justify patient´s expenses for treatment performance.

Introduction

Sweating is a physiological process, ensuring homeostasis of thermoregulation. The core temperature of the body should be constantly between 36.3 and 37.4°C. [1] During coldness muscles are trembling and blood vessels are contracting in order to reduce the outward flow of heat. If core temperature is increased the sympathicus activates eccrine sweat glands producing sweat by using this heat as heat of vaporization. [2] The eccrine sweat glands are innervated by cholinergic fibres and they are distributed all over the body surface. They are concentrated at palms, soles, axillaries, forehead and back. The overall number is estimated to be 3-4 millions on skin (about 5% are active at the same time), with a mean density of 300/cm^2. [3, 4]

Hyperhidrosis is a disorder of excessive sweating beyond what is physiologically necessary for thermoregulation. [5] Primary focal hyperhidrosis is the most common type of overactive sweating. Due to the unknown cause it´s also called “idiopathic”, “essential” or “genuine” hyperhidrosis. “Primary” means, that no other exo- or endogenous cause is obvious for overactive sweating and “focal” means, that the hyperhidrosis is located in a defined area. Primary focal hyperhidrosis has an extremely impact on well-being, especially on occupational, physical, emotional and social life of patients. [6, 7] Therefore, health-related quality of life has been developed as core outcomes parameter on treatment. [8, 9] As the amount of sweating underlies a huge interpersonal variability, fixed thresholds for quantity of sweat per time are only a point of orientation. [10] Much more important is the individual rating of patients quality of life.

Within this paper we want to review current available epidemiological knowledge on hyperhidrosis, the recommendations of guidelines on therapy and the validity of quality of life questionnaires. But as hyperhidrosis treatment often has to be paid by patients themselves, we want to focus on the pay for performance. Which therapy shows the best cost-effectiveness, whereof outcomes have been measured with quality of life instruments? And does this have any consequences on the decision-making process of patients and physicians?

Methods

Epidemiology

Epidemiological studies to hyperhidrosis have been identified after a literature research in PubMed on 18th of March 2014. The term "hyperhidrosis" was combined with either "epidemiology", "prevalence" or "incidence". Only original papers published (in English or German) on human subjects, investigating adults and adolescents with a formal diagnosis of hyperhidrosis combined with a prevalence or incidence rate have been considered.

Guidelines

Current evidence based guidelines or recommendations on the treatment of focal hyperhidrosis published between January 2005 and May 2014 have been identified by literature research in Guideline International Network, AWMF, National Guideline Clearinghouse, PubMed and specific guideline provider like dermatological associations within the internet using the term: "hyperhidrosis" in combination with "guideline" or "recommendation". References of the papers initially extracted were also searched to identify more guidelines. All identified papers have been reviewed for the previously defined inclusion criteria and additionally for the issue if patient reported outcomes data have had an impact on the recommendation, the guideline offers.

Quality of Life Instruments

To identify instruments used in HRQol assessment in hyperhidrosis a literature search was done in PubMed, PsycINFO and EMBASE. The initial search was based on the following terms: "hyperhidrosis and quality of life"; "hyperhidrosis and daily life"; "hyperhidrosis and clinical trial"; "hyperhidrosis and impact". References of the papers initially extracted were also searched to identify more material for our review. An additional search strategy was based on the identified instrument e.g. "SF-36 and hyperhidrosis", "DLQI and hyperhidrosis".

A study was included if it reported the application of a HRQol instrument in hyperhidrosis patients or if it reported the psychometric properties of the instrument. An instrument was included if it was developed for the measurement of HRQol (or its components) and if it had been used in hyperhidrosis patients. Such instruments could be disease specific, dermatology -specific or generic. We limited ourselves to HRQoL self-assessed by patients, either self-completed questionnaire or interviewer administered.

Information related to the instruments was extracted following standard quality criteria for HRQoL instruments. [11, 12] Information extracted included key psychometric properties, descriptive information and additionally details of studies applying the instrument. See Appendix 1 for the data extraction form used.

Quality of Life As an Outcome Parameter

For identifying studies with quality of life as an outcome parameter, a literature search in PubMed was performed with a combination of the term "*axillary hyperhidrosis*" and the following terms: *Aluminium Chloride, Botulinum Toxin, surgery, ETS, oxybutynin, Methantheline, bornaprine, iontophoresis, sage, HDSS, DLQI, QoL and quality of life*.

On 30th of July 2013, 577 studies have been identified and reviewed for the a priori defined inclusion and exclusion criteria. The studies should include research on human subjects exclusively, investigating adults and adolescents with a formal diagnosis of axillary hyperhidrosis, evaluating treatment which is recommended in German National Guideline for Hyperhidrosis, (randomized) controlled studies with at least 4 weeks of observation period and with detailed information of drug exposition to patients. Studies in English or German that evaluated discrete values of HDSS and/or DLQI as outcomes for patients with axillary hyperhidrosis have been included. Excluded were studies evaluating treatment options, which are not available in Germany, studies with less than 12 patients per treatment group, dose finding studies, case reports and case studies. Moreover responder rates for HRQoL instruments often are used within clinical trials. A responder is defined e.g. as a patient with a reduction of 2 points in HDSS. Even if such dichotomic outcomes allow a simple scoring, it does not reflect the complexity of quality of life development under therapy. Therefore we decided to use differences of means for outcomes values in order to value the power of improvement of each therapy.

Treatment and Drug Costs

As HRQoL for hyperhidrosis treatment is evaluated commonly over short-time period, the utility model covers a timeframe of only 4 weeks. Nevertheless, overall treatment costs have been modeled for a period of 2 years. The cost considered for hyperhidrosis drugs were the manufacturer's selling price stated in the German Catalogue of Pharmaceutical Specialties plus VAT. Treatment costs have been calculated according German Medical Fee Index (GOA), considering consultation, examination and Minor´s test for the first visit of each treatment and if applicable, intradermal injection 10 or 15 times on each axillae (GOA Numbers 1, 5, 252 and 752). It has been assumed, that Minor´s test will be performed once a year. For patients with systemic treatment, a visit every three month and monthly drug costs have been assumed; for topical treatment a visit every three months and drug costs either every or every second month have been assumed. Minimum treatment costs for injectable drugs consider consultation, examination, Minor´s test and 10 injections every 12 months, maximum treatment costs consider consultation, examination, Minor´s test and 15 injections every 6 months. All prizes have been calculated in Euros, US$ prizes have been calculated into Euros according exchange rate (27.04.2014) of 1US$=0.7722€.

Results

Epidemiology

In total, 209 studies have been identified, whereof 9 contained relevant information to prevalence or incidence to hyperhidrosis (see table 1).

Table 1. Epidemiological studies on hyperhidrosis with prevalence or incidence rates for axillary and palmar hyperhidrosis and overall prevalence or incidence

Study	Hyperhidrosis prevalence	Axillary hyperhidrosis prevalence	Palmar hyperhidrosis prevalence	Hyperhidrosis incidence
Stefaniak et al. 2013	16.7%			
Augustin et al. 2013	16.3%	7.2%		
Fujimoto et al. 2013		5.75%		
Westphal et al. 2011	5.5%	1.25%		
Chu et al. 2010				7.2 per 10.000
Felini et al. 2009	9.0%			
Li et al. 2007			4.36%	
Tu et al. 2007			4.59%	
Strutton et al. 2004	2.8%	1.4 %		

Strutton et al. investigated the prevalence of hyperhidrosis and the impact on individuals in the US with special focus on axillary hyperhidrosis. [13] For this survey 150,000 US households were screened and all necessary data (e.g. age, sex of all members) were collected to extrapolate to the general US population. The Hyperhidrosis Disease Severity Scale (HDSS) and the Hyperhidrosis Impact Questionnaire (HHIQ) were used for evaluation. The survey showed that 2.8% of the US population suffered from hyperhidrosis whereas the rate between male (2.9%) and female responders (2.8%) was similar. The effect of hyperhidrosis was most pronounced in the working population at the age of 25 to 64 years and lowest at the age under 12 years with 3.5-4.5% and 0.5-0.7%, respectively. Only 38% of the affected persons discussed their problem with a health care specialist whereas the rate for females was higher than for males with 47.5% and 28.6%, respectively. Approximately half of the people who suffered from hyperhidrosis had axillary hyperhidrosis that means about 1.4% of the US population. Among these individuals 32.4% had problems with sweating which affected the daily life extremely. The impairment was particularily observed in the working productivity and as well in the psychical, social and physical sectors.

To obtain more detailed epidemiological data from Germany Augustin et al. performed a study with 51 German companies of different branches including 14,336 individuals between the age of 16 to 70. [14] A dermatological screening program for skin cancer was used for investigation – added by epidemiological questions to hyperhidrosis. [15, 16] The overall prevalence of hyperhidrosis in this representative population was 16.3% whereas the illness was more pronounced in males than in females, with 18.1% and 13.3 %, respectively. From individuals who reported hyperhidrosis 68% suffered from generalized and 28% from focal hyperhidrosis. Most affected areas were the axillaries (44%) followed by feet (29%) and hands (23%; others 34%). For 77.5% of individuals with hyperhidrosis the disease was a burden and influenced their daily activities.

Prevalence data from Japan have been provided by Fujimoto et al. who performed a questionnaire survey for people aged 5-64 in 2013. In total, 5807 valid responses showed prevalence rates of 5.33% for primary palm hyperhidrosis, 2.79% for primary plantar hyperhidrosis, 5.75% for primary axillary hyperhidrosis and 4.7% for primary head hyperhidrosis. [17]

In a recent epidemiological study Westphal et al. estimate the prevalence of primary hyperhidrosis among 293 students of the Faculty of Medicine, in Manaus to 5.5%. [18]

The prevalence of hyperhidrosis among young Polish adults was evaluated by Stefaniak et al. in 2013. Forty-two (16.7%) out of 253 participants declared that they suffer from hyperhidrosis. [19]

The incidence on hyperhidrosis palmaris in Taiwan in 2004, based on secondary data analysis by Taiwan's National Health Insurance database was detected to 7.2 per 10,000 beneficiaries. In total, 15,839 patients with hyperhidrosis palmaris were identified. The incidence was highest among patients aged 20-29 years old and higher among female than male (7.4 vs. 6.9 per 10.000 beneficiaries). [20]

Among 500 randomly selected subjects in Blumenau, Brazil, 45 patients could be identified with primary hyperhidrosis by utilizing interviews. This refers to a prevalence rate of 9.0%, whereof a greater prevalence could be identified among men (10.62%) than among women (7.66%). [21]

Among 33 000 college and high school students (15-22 years old) in three cities of southeast China a prevalence rate of 4.36% for primary palmar hyperhidrosis could be identified. [22] Primary palmar hyperhidrosis in adolescent in Fuzhou was seen with a comparable prevalence of 4.59% affecting both sexes equally. [23]

Guidelines

Ten out of 24 recommendations or guidelines on hyperhidrosis treatment fulfilled the above mentioned criteria (see table 2).

Table 2. Recommendations or guidelines on treatment of hyperhidrosis

Author	Title	Country
Perera et al.	Hyperhidrosis and bromhidrosis -- a guide to assessment and management.	Australia
Walling et al.	Treatment options for hyperhidrosis.	USA
Cerfolio et al.	The Society of Thoracic Surgeons expert consensus for the surgical treatment of hyperhidrosis	USA
Moreno Balsalobre et al.	Guidelines on surgery of the thoracic sympathetic nervous system	Spain
Hölzle et al.	Recommendations for tap water iontophoresis	Germany
Solish et al.	A comprehensive approach to the recognition, diagnosis, and severity-based treatment of focal hyperhidrosis: recommendations of the Canadian Hyperhidrosis Advisory Committee.	Canada
Wörle et al.	Definition and treatment of primary hyperhidrosis	Germany
De Campos et al.	Treatment options for primary hyperhidrosis.	Brazil
Hoorens et al.	Primary focal hyperhidrosis: current treatment options and a step-by-step approach.	Belgium
Gelbard et al.	Primary pediatric hyperhidrosis: a review of current treatment options.	USA

All of them recommend a step-by-step approach of interventions. Pharmacological treatments of focal hyperhidrosis include topical, oral and iontophoretic treatments as well as Botulinum Toxin A injections. Surgical interventions like suction curettage appear to be an effective and relatively safe treatment for axillary hyperhidrosis before stepping up to sympathetic denervation which is seen generally as the last step in treating severe palmar, craniofacial and axillary hyperhidrosis. [24]

Patients with focal hyperhidrosis present most often bilateral an excessive sweating of the axillae, hands, soles or the face. Generally all guidelines recommend firstly the use of topical treatment with Aluminium Chloride. Different vehicles are used, as ethyl alcohol-(water-solution), salicylic acid gel or thermophobic foams. Only some authors recommend the supportive use of topical corticoids, like hydrocortisone, in case of hypersensitivity or irritation due to $AlCl_3$. [25]

Walling et al. recommend topical treatment as first-line treatment for axillary and palmoplantar hyperhidrosis. For axillary hyperhidrosis, Botulinum Toxin injections are suggested as second-line treatment, systemic treatment as third-line treatment, local surgery as fourth-line treatment, and endoscopic thoracic sympathectomy as fifth-line treatment. Systemic treatment with glycopyrrolate or clonidine should be considered as second line treatment for palmar and plantar hyperhidrosis. [26]

In contrast to the above mentioned recommendations, the Society of Thoracic Surgeons' General Thoracic Workforce suggests, that primary hyperhidrosis of the extremities, axillae or face should be best treated by endoscopic thoracic sympathectomy. [27]

The "Guidelines on surgery of the thoracic sympathetic nervous system" by Moreno Balsalobre et al. recommend high concentration of Aluminium Chloride as the topical treatment of choice. In parallel Botulinum Toxin A is seen as very effective in the control of axillary hyperhidrosis. The authors rate the results as "not as good in patients with palmar hyperhidrosis and of little use in plantar and craniofacial hyperhidrosis". [28]

A specialized guideline on the treatment of focal hyperhidrosis with tap-water iontophoresis was published by Hölzle et al. The aim of this guideline was to optimize safety and success rate by introducing standardized procedures. The authors especially focus on the technical data of the devices and the standardized performance of treatment according diagnosis, including follow-up to track quality of the results. [29]

Perera et al. specially recommend the use of glycopyrrolate iontophoresis instead of less effective tap-water iontophoresis. In their opinion propantheline bromide and oxybutynin are the most common anticholinergics used. [25] Moreover they express, that surgery is reserved for those patients who are refractory to medical therapy.

During a consensus meeting, the Canadian Hyperhidrosis Advisory Committee designed an algorithm of treatment according severity and location of hyperhidrosis. Starting point is the self-evaluation of patient's burden of disease according HDSS. As recommended in other guidelines, mild axillary, palmar, and plantar hyperhidrosis (HDSS 1 or 2) should initially be treated with topical Aluminum Chloride, followed by Botulinum Toxin A and iontophoresis (palmar, plantar) as second-line treatment. For severe cases of axillary, palmar and plantar hyperhidrosis (HDSS 3 or 4) Botulinum Toxin A and topical Aluminium Chloride is seen as first line treatment. For craniofacial hyperhidrosis Botulinum Toxin A, topical Aluminium Chloride and systemic anticholinergics and for plantar and palmar hyperhidrosis, iontophoresis is recommended as first line treatment. Surgery and ETS is only recommended in case of failure of all other treatment options. [30]

The German AWMF guideline on treatment of primary hyperhidrosis offers a comparable armentarium of step-by-step procedures for treatment. [10] (see table 3)

Table 3. Therapy modalities for axillary, palmar and generalized hyperhidrosis (adapted from German AWMF guideline on treatment of primary hyperhidrosis)

Axillary hyperhidrosis
1. topical therapy with antiperspirants
2. chemical denervation with Botulinum Toxin A
3. surgical sweat gland excision
4. systemic therapy with antiperspirants or psychotropic drugs
Palmar and plantar hyperhidrosis
1. topical therapy with antiperspirants
2. tap-water iontophoresis
3. chemical denervation with Botulinum Toxin A
4. systemic therapy with antiperspirants or psychotropic drugs
5. ultima ratio: thoracic sympathectomy
Generalized hyperhidrosis
1. systemic therapy with antiperspirants or psychotropic drugs

Quality of Life Instruments

Description of Instruments

Full descriptive details are available in Table 4. Five instruments assess disease specific HRQol (dsQol), four assess dermatology specific HRQol (dmQol) and the remaining four assess generic HRQol (HRQol). On the other hand, the instruments focus on slightly differing concepts, with only a few providing a broader coverage of Qol. For instance the HHIQ, HDSS and DLQI concentrate on impairment in daily life activities, while instruments like the PBI and IIRS might be said to assess rather even more distinct concepts, 'patient therapeutic benefit' and 'lifestyle disruption', respectively. Except for HHIQ, all dsQol instruments target a specific sub-group of HH patients, for instance the HQLQ, HQ, and HS were developed for use in patients treated with ETS surgery. The HDSS which has had wider usage in various patient sub-groups was developed for axillary HH patients. On the other hand, the dmQol and HRQol instruments reviewed are versatile in terms of their target populations, patient with various (dermatologic – in the case of dmQol) conditions were involved in their development. Noteworthy still is that among these, only the PBI included hyperhidrosis patients in its development. Both, the PBI and the FLQA applied a more inclusive approach in their item generation without limiting their samples to patients seeking for treatment at clinics.

Among the dsQol measures only the HQ has a formally confirmed structure; based on factor analysis. For the dmQol measures only the structure of the PBI and the Skindex are supported by evidence. [31] Available literature on the DLQI has yielded mixed conclusions on its structure (ibid). The dimensions and structure of all gQoL are adequately supported.

Psychometric Properties

The psychometric properties of each instrument were evaluated. Each property was classified as strong (++), moderate (+), poor (-), information not provided (0) or not applicable (n.a.) based on recommended review standards and criteria and presented in table 5. [11] Aaronson et al. propose eight attributes as a basis for reviewing instruments, including: conceptual measurement model, reliability, validity, responsiveness, interpretability, respondent and administrative burden, alternative forms, cultural and language adaptations, this review focuses on the first six.

Table 4. Descriptive properties of instruments

Questionnaire (Refs.)	Target Population	Concept Assessed	No. of Scales	No. of Items	Response options	Range of Scores
HHIQ	Primary focal HH	daily life impairment	-	41-baseline; 10- follow up	Varies	-
HDSS	Primary axillary HH	dubjective disease severity; daily life impairment	1	1	Likert type; 4	1-4
HS	ETS treated palmar-plantar HH patients	Physical Symptoms & Social impairment	1	15	Likert type; 10	0 -150
HQ	Surgically treated HH patients	disease specific HRQoL	5	34	Likert type; 5	34 -170
HQLQ	Outpatients awaiting for surgery	disease Specific HRQoL – daily life impairment	-	20	Likert type; 5	20 - 100
FLQA	Dermatology patients	Dermatology - HRQoL	6	46 plus 3 VAS	5 plus	NA
DLQI	Dermatology patients	Dermatology-HRQoL	-	10	Likert type; 4	0 -30
Skindex-29	Dermatology patients	Dermatology-HRQoL	3	30	Likert type; 5	0 - 100
PBI	Dermatologic patients incl. HH	Therapeutic benefit	5	23	Likert type; 5	0-4
SF-36	General population	HR-QoL	8	36	Varies	0 - 100
SF-12	General population	HR-QoL	8	12	Varies	0 -100
NHP	General population	HR-QoL	6	38	2	0-100
IIRS	Chronic illness patients	disease severity (Illness intrusiveness)	3	13	7	13 -91

Validity

The accuracy of conclusions made based on an instrument depends on its validity i.e. the ability of the instrument to measure what it was intended to measure. [32] This is reflected in various forms of validity including content and construct validity. Content validity relates to the evidence supporting the appropriateness of domains and items of the instrument vis-à-vis the intended use. [11] This can be demonstrated via involvement of target population in item generation and the involvement of experts to the relevance of the content.

Out of all instruments reviewed, only the HQLQ showed inadequate validity in its content. Its developers report that they were inspired by a previous Qol instrument. [33] The DLQI and Skindex report involvement of patients attending dermatologic clinic and private practice respectively. FLQA and PBI report open surveys of patients and interviews as basis for their items. Although the dsQol and HRQol meet the requisite criteria, lack of involvement of HH patients in the former and dermatologic patients in the latter is a disadvantage. Among these two classes of instruments, the PBI and IIRS have been validated in HH patients. Another aspect of validity – 'construct validity' relates to extent to which proposed interpretation of scores (hypotheses) based on theoretical implications associated with underlying constructs being measured is supported. [11] Various techniques including factor analysis, known-groups validation, and convergence/discriminant validity are often used. [34] The HQLQ provided inadequate evidence for the validity of its construct in contrast to two other dsQol instruments, the HHIQ and HDSS which reported strong evidence. Evidence for the HS and HQ reflected a moderate form of construct validity. Factor analysis was applied only in one dsQol (the HQ).

Except for FLQA rated moderately, all dmQol measures showed strong construct validity, based on multiple methods. The convergence of FLQA to comparable scales of existing instruments, the DLQI and ALLTAG questionnaires showed a rather moderate correlation. The validity of HRQol instruments is supported by various forms of evidence including hypothesis testing, known-groups validation as well as correlations with other validated instruments.

Reliability

Another requisite property of a Qol instrument is that its measurements are reliable i.e. reproducible and free from random error. [65] In classical test theory, reliability is assessed through analyzing 'internal consistency' and 'reproducibility' (test-retest and inter-observer) of the instrument. [11] The former reflects the extent to which items are inter-related [34] and is often assessed using 'Cronbach Alpha coefficient' or 'Kuder-Richardson formula 20', both of which are measures of correlation in multi-item scales.

Only the HQ reported evidence for internal consistency among the dsQol while it is inapplicable for the HDSS (a single item scale). Only the FLQA and NHP had less than strong internal consistency for the rest of the instruments reviewed. None of the dsQol reported test-retest reliability except for the HDSS. On the other hand the rest of the instruments, except for the PBI, reported robust test-retest reproducibility. The PBI showed only moderate test-retest reliability based on partial correlations ($r = 0.68$) tested after 4 to 8 weeks.

Table 5. Psychometric properties of quality of life questionnaires used for hyperhidrosis treatment

Questionnaire	Content Validity	Construct Validity	Convergent Validity	Internal Consistency	Test-Retest Reliability	Responsiveness	Floor & Ceiling effects	Inter - pretability	MCID	Respondent Burden	Structure
Disease Specific HRQol instruments											
HHIQ[35-37]	++	++	++	++	0	0	++	0	0	0	0
HDSS[38-41]	++	++	++	na	++	++	0	+	+	++	na
HS[42]	++	++	+	++	0	++	0	+	0	0	na
HQ[43]	++	+	0	++	0	0	0	0	0	++	+
HQLQ[44-46]	-	-	0	0	0	-	0	0	0	0	0
Dermatology HRQol Specific Questionnaire											
FLQA[47, 48]	++	++	+	+	++	++	+	++	0	0	0
DLQI) [49-51]	++	++	++	++	+	++	+	++	++	++	-

Questionnaire	Content Validity	Construct Validity	Convergent Validity	Internal Consistency	Test-Retest Reliability	Responsiveness	Floor & Ceiling effects	Inter - pretability	MCID	Respondent Burden	Structure
Skindex[51-58]	++	++	++	++	++	++	++	++	0	+	+
PBI[31, 59, 60]	++	++	+	++	+	+	+	+	0	0	+
Generic HRQol Questionnaire											
SF-36) [57, 61]	++	++	++	++	++	++	+	+	++	+	+
SF-12[61]	++	++	++	++	++	+	++	+		++	+
NHP[61]	++	++	++	+	++	+	+	0	0	++	+
IIRS[62] [63, 64]	+	++	++	++	++	++	0	0	0	0	+

Note: While Teale, Roberts et al. 2002 claim that the HHIQ has favourable internal consistency, test-retest reliability, construct and convergent validity, the relevant correlations were not reported.

Responsiveness

Another requisite property, particularly for evaluative instruments, is the ability to detect changes in the construct of interest, experienced by a given patient, over time. [11] Measuring responsiveness can be done by testing hypothesis, following two main approaches; the first option centers around estimating an effect size statistic; the other approach compares the t-statistic of one instrument with that of a related instrument to produce a ratio e.g. relative efficiency. [34]

Only the HDSS was rated as having strong responsiveness among the dsQol. Although the other dsQol measures like HHIQ, HS, HQLQ reported significant changes in item scores following treatment, they were rated moderately due to the methodology followed. The Skindex and DLQI demonstrated evidence for strong responsiveness, the FLQA and the PBI reflected a moderate degree of responsiveness owing the same factors as dsQol measures. The SF-36, SF-12, NHP, IIRS were rated as having strong responsiveness, based on evidence from other disease conditions. As a caveat, the responsiveness of generic measures in HH patients, relative to disease specific or dermatologic specific measures, would be expected to be moderate [66] confirmed this for SF-36 and HS.

Table 6. Hyperhidrosis Disease Severity Scale

HDSS questionaire
'How would you rate the severity of your hyperhidrosis?'
• My sweating is never noticeable and never interferes with my daily activities: 1
• My sweating is tolerable but sometimes interferes with my daily activities: 2
• My sweating is barely tolerable and frequently interferes with my daily activities: 3
• My sweating is intolerable and always interferes with my daily activities: 4
Score of 1: mild; Score of 2: moderate; Score of 3–4: severe.

Interpretation of Scores

Only the HDSS and HS reported data to aid interpretation of results among the dsQoL, in the form of distribution based cut-offs. All dmQoL have a form of interpretation supportive data; anchor based in the case of DLQI and Skindex; distribution based in the case of FLQA. The IIRS was the only gQoL with no form of interpretation data available. MCID is reported for the DLQI, SF-36 and SF-12 only.

Measurement Model

No sufficient information has been reported on the distribution of scores for all dsQol measures. Only Skindex has the highest rating i.e. no floor or ceiling effects. The other instruments, SF-36, SF-12, NHP, IIRS, and DLQI were rated moderately. The FLQA and PBI both received a poor rating as floor/ceiling effect were in excess of 20%.

Structure

Excluding the HDSS, a single item measure, evaluation of the dimensions was not reported for all dsQol measures and the FLQA. Factor analyses were reported for the rest of the instruments, although studies on the DLQI are in disagreement over the number of factors, ranging from 1 to 4. [49] Information on fit with Rasch model has also been reported for SF-36, SF-12, NHP, DLQI and Skindex. It is noteworthy that none of the instruments fit the Rasch model indisputably.

Treatment and Drug Costs

Out of 577 studies only 3 papers with 4 different treatment modalities could be identified, fulfilling the inclusion and exclusion criteria. (see table 7) Patients have been treated with either 150 mg Methantheline per day, topical Aluminium Chloride (thin layer, without occlusion to clean, dry axilla nightly), 50 U or 75 U Botulinum Toxin A once by a parallel evaluation of quality of life with HDSS and/or DLQI.

The drug costs for Methantheline per month was 51.48 €, for Aluminium Chloride 15.01€ or 17.31€, for 50 U Botulinum Toxin A minimum 164.12€ or maximum 203.44€ and for 75 U Botulinum Toxin A minimum 328.23€ or maximum 406.87€. Drug costs cover the period of 2 years, presented in figure 1. The minimum prize for Aluminium Chloride, followed by the minimum prize for 50 U Botulinum Toxin A could be identified as cheapest drugs. Methantheline and 75 U of Botulinum Toxin A with maximum prize used each 6 months could be identified as the most expensive drugs.

Adding the treatment cost for consultation (21.44€), Minors-Test (40.22€) at least once a year and injections (53.60 for 10 injections or 80.40€ for 15 injections) to the above mentioned drug costs, the overall treatment with 50 U Botulinum Toxin A with minimum prize is the cheapest treatment over a two year period (416.08 €) (see table 8).

Table 7. Randomized studies on treatment of axillary hyperhidrosis with DLQI and/or HDSS as outcomes criteria

Reference	No of patients	Study type	Observation period	Medicinal Product	Drug	Dose	DLQI Baseline	DLQI at follow-up	DLQI Delta	HDSS baseline	HDSS at follow-up	HDSS Delta
Müller et al. 2012	128	randomized, placebo-controlled trial	4 weeks	Vagantin	Methantheline	150 mg per day	16.6	9.7 on day 28 ± 1	6.9	3.2	2.4 on day 28 ± 1	0.8
Flanagan et al.	22	single-center, randomized, open-label	4, 8 and 12 weeks	Botox	Botulinum Toxin A	50 U of Botox per axilla				3.63	1.21 at week 4;	2.42
Flanagan et al.	23	single-center, randomized, open-label	4, 8 and 12 weeks	Drysol	20% Aluminium Chloride	thin layer of AC				3.71	2.38 at week 4	1.33
Lowe et al.	102	multicenter, double-blind, randomized, placebo-controlled, parallel-group study	4 weeks	Botox	Botulinum Toxin A	75 per axilla	9.3	2.1	7.2	3.5		
Lowe et al.	94	multicenter, double-blind, randomized, placebo-controlled, parallel-group study	4 weeks	Botox	Botulinum Toxin A	50 U per axilla	7.8	2.2	5.6	3.5		

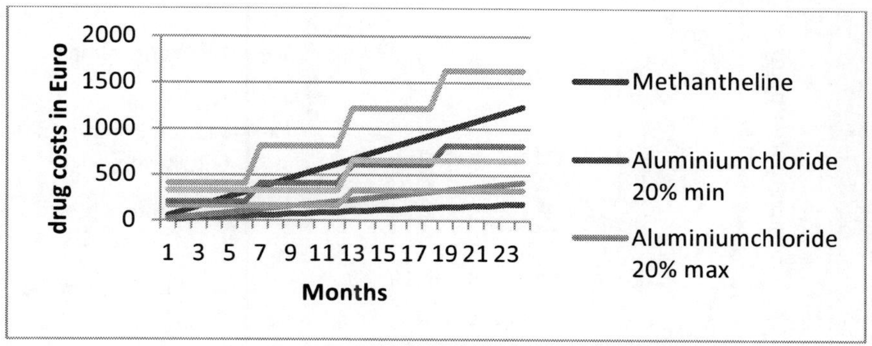

Figure 1. Drug costs model for hyperhidrosis treatment for Methantheline, Aluminium Chloride and Botulinum Toxin A over a 2 year period.

Table 8. Hyperhidrosis treatment cost model for treatment with Methantheline, Aluminiumchloride and Botulinum Toxin A over a 2 year period

Month	Methan-theline	Aluminium Chloride 20% min	Aluminium Chloride 20% max	50 U Botulinum Toxin min	50 U Botulinum Toxin max	75 U Botulinum Toxin min	75 U Botulinum Toxin max
1	123,86	87,39	89,69	290,1	356,22	454,21	559,65
2	175,34	87,39	107	290,1	356,22	454,21	559,65
3	226,82	102,4	124,31	290,1	356,22	454,21	559,65
4	299,74	123,84	163,06	290,1	356,22	454,21	559,65
5	351,22	138,85	180,37	290,1	356,22	454,21	559,65
6	402,7	138,85	197,68	290,1	356,22	454,21	559,65
7	475,62	175,3	236,43	290,1	712,44	454,21	1119,3
8	527,1	175,3	253,74	290,1	712,44	454,21	1119,3
9	578,58	190,31	271,05	290,1	712,44	454,21	1119,3
10	651,5	211,75	309,8	290,1	712,44	454,21	1119,3
11	702,98	226,76	327,11	290,1	712,44	454,21	1119,3
12	754,46	226,76	344,42	290,1	712,44	454,21	1119,3
13	878,32	314,15	434,11	416,08	1068,66	908,42	1678,95
14	929,8	314,15	451,42	416,08	1068,66	908,42	1678,95
15	981,28	329,16	468,73	416,08	1068,66	908,42	1678,95
16	1054,2	350,6	507,48	416,08	1068,66	908,42	1678,95
17	1105,68	365,61	524,79	416,08	1068,66	908,42	1678,95
18	1157,16	365,61	542,1	416,08	1068,66	908,42	1678,95
19	1230,08	402,06	580,85	416,08	1424,88	908,42	2238,6
20	1281,56	402,06	598,16	416,08	1424,88	908,42	2238,6
21	1333,04	417,07	615,47	416,08	1424,88	908,42	2238,6
22	1405,96	438,51	654,22	416,08	1424,88	908,42	2238,6
23	1457,44	453,52	671,53	416,08	1424,88	908,42	2238,6
24	1508,92	453,52	688,84	416,08	1424,88	908,42	2238,6

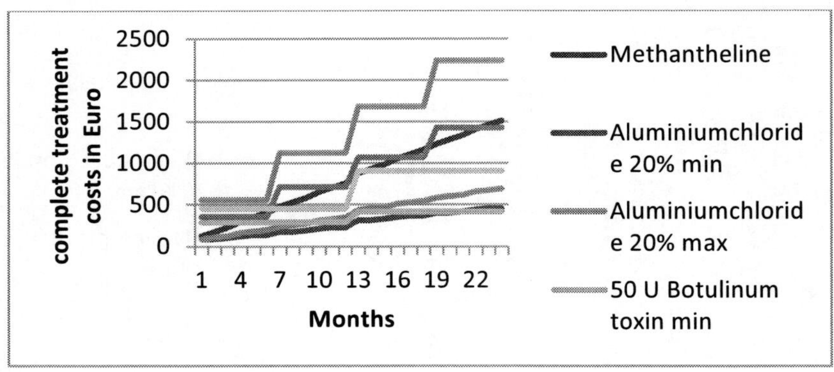

Figure 2. Hyperhidrosis treatment cost model for treatment with Methantheline, Aluminiumchloride and Botulinum Toxin A over a 2 year period.

By calculating the Delta DLQI and Delta HDSS, shown in table 7, and the overall treatment cost for a 4-week treatment time, the cost per DLQI and cost per HDSS could be calculated. Using the DLQI as outcome criteria the overall treatment costs to improve one point on DLQI is lowest with Methantheline treatment (17.95€). Using HDSS as HRQoL questionnaire, Aluminium Chloride min showed the best cost-effectiveness with 65,71€ per 1 point improvement. (see table 9)

Table 9. Cost-effectiveness model calculation the costs per improvement of 1 point on DLQI or HDSS

	Delta DLQI	Delta HDSS	Costs per 4 weeks	costs per DLQI	costs per HDSS
Methantheline	6,9	0,8	123,86	17,95	154,83
AlCl3 min		1,33	87,39		65,71
AlCl3 max		1,33	89,69		67,44
50 U Botox min	5,6	2,42	290,1	51,80	119,88
50 U Botox max	5,6	2,42	356,22	63,61	147,20
75 U Botox min	7,2		454,21	63,08	
75 U Botox max	7,2		559,65	77,73	

Discussion

Epidemiology

This review provides a detailed overview of the existing data on the worldwide incidence and prevalence of hyperhidrosis. The results from the review confirmed that hyperhidrosis is a common disease; prevalence rates showed a worldwide geographic variation that probably reflects the fact that hyperhidrosis is a complex disease influenced by both autonomous nervous system and environmental factors.

Since Struttons publication in 2004, all new epidemiological studies on hyperhidrosis showed higher prevalence rates. This reflects either the increased awareness of sweating or the increased use of patient reported outcomes instruments, reflecting the burden of disease on validated scales. We therefore strongly appreciate Augustin et al. data using a representative sample size (for German population) and investigating patient's health status exclusively by dermatologists. [14] By doing so, a dramatic higher quality of data and in parallel a higher prevalence rate of hyperhidrosis in general but also of all subgroups could be identified. Epidemiological studies are an important contributor to our understanding of hyperhidrosis, and there is a need for future international research collaborations using standardized methodology to address knowledge gaps that still exist on the disease and potential trends in prevalence and incidence over time.

Guidelines

In general, the recommendations of the guidelines on diagnosis, assessment and non-/pharmacological management were consistent. Performance of Minors starch iodine test was recommended as the mainstay for the diagnosis of hyperhidrosis. Across the guidelines, major differences were only recognized between guidelines presented by a surgical association [27] and all others authors, related to recommendations of either pharmacological or surgical management. All, except Cerfolio et al., follow a step-by-step approach presented by Hoorens et al. [24] Topical Aluminium Chloride is seen generally as first line treatment for focal hyperhidrosis. On second step, guidelines present different recommendations on the use of Botulinum Toxin A, iontophoresis, systemic anticholinergics and surgical interventions. Nevertheless, for generalized hyperhidrosis, the recommendations are consistent, proposing systemic acting drugs. HDSS is recognized as the qualitative QoL instrument of choice. [10, 24] The reflection of duration of treatment effect, side effects, any complications, costs, local level of availability of health care and patient wishes for treatment are additional factors which are partly implemented but should be much more extended within guidelines of focal hyperhidrosis.

Quality of Life Instruments

A total of 13 instruments were identified through a comprehensive literature search via databases and a manual search of references of identified articles. The majority of instruments identified were disease specific (5 out of 13), followed by an equal number of dermatology specific (n = 4) and generic instruments (n =4). The number of disease specific instruments is comparable to available disease specific measures for psoriasis (n = 4) and acne (n = 4) based on corresponding reviews. [67]; [68] Previous reviews of quality of life measures in hyperhidrosis have found up to eight instruments, moreover, psychometric properties of the measures were not appraised in both reviews. [69, 70]

Although all generic instruments have been validated in other patient populations besides their application in clinical research in hyperhidrosis patients, only the IIRS had a study evaluating its psychometric properties in hyperhidrosis patients. [64] Among the dermatology specific instruments, only the PBI and DLQI have known psychometric properties in hyperhidrosis patients. In particular, the DLQI has been used as a reference tool for validation of other QOL instruments for hyperhidrosis e.g. HDSS and HHIQ. [35, 36]

Concerning methodological quality, there were inadequacies reflected in the design and method of evaluation of construct validity and responsiveness, which has equally been noted in other conditions e.g. in a review of Osteoarthritis Questionnaires by Veenhof et al. [71] Clear hypotheses were not set ex-ante, for the majority of instruments, despite the studies showing a significant difference in scores ex-post as basis for construct validity. Among the disease specific instruments only HQ utilised factor analysis. Likewise for responsiveness, standard measures were not reported in all disease specific instruments; in its place a claim of responsiveness was based on statistical significance of the change in scores. There is a noticeable use of ad-hoc instruments, un-validated, in the assessment of quality of life in surgically treated hyperhidrosis patients, especially in studies evaluating the surgically treated patients. [72] Such instruments were excluded from this review for their lack of psychometric information.

Choice of optimal instrument for research in hyperhidrosis has to reflect among others, the purpose of the research and the intended target population. [57] The HDSS is the instrument of choice, with a caveat of being ill-suited for capturing the full-profile of health status of patients. Among the generic instruments the IIRS would be the most preferred, again with the downside of poor interpretability of results. The major drawback with the other generic instruments e.g. SF-36, NHP is that they include items which have no relevance to hyperhidrosis patients. This is not to say that such differences in sensitivity between disease specific instruments and generic instruments are non-existent in other disease conditions, but rather that the magnitude of such differences may actually compromise study results in hyperhidrosis.

Treatment Costs in Decision Making Process

Even if each treatment option has its justification in the armentarium of hyperhidrosis treatment, the modalities of application, duration of effect and absolute effect of improvement are varying extremely. The oral anticholingergic Methantheline needs an application three times a day. Depending on its pharmacokinetic profile, Methantheline is slowly absorbed and rapidly eliminated in humans. Methanthelines inhibitory effect is closely associated with its plasma concentrations following a standard sigmoid pharmacodynamic model. [73] Aluminium chloride also needs a regular application. Depending on the tolerability of dose and formulation, it differs between daily and three times a week. [74, 75] Only Botulinum Toxin A is generally injected once every 3 to 12 months. [76, 77] It's the only drug which shows significant increase in the duration of efficacy with the repetition of injections in patients with primary palmar and axillary hyperhidrosis. [78, 79]

As hyperhidrosis is a permanent disorder, a cost-effectiveness model over a longer period would be useful. Unfortunately there are no outcomes data available reflecting this issue. We therefore increased the model to evaluate drug costs and treatment costs within 24 months. Aluminium Chloride seems to be the cheapest drug, the therapy with 50 U Botulinum Toxin A min the cheapest treatment and Methantheline showed the best cost-effectiveness, when DLQI was used as patient reported outcome.

As in Germany not every hyperhidrosis treatment is paid by health insurances. Most often Botulinum Toxin A therapy has to be paid by patients themselves. The comparison between costs was therefore explicitly done on patient's perspective – as costs and outcomes would both affect patient's decision for treatment.

So far, we could not observe any study, which includes any patient reported outcomes into the decision making process of any guideline or recommendation. So what could be the consequences for dermatologists? Does pay-for-performance plays a relevant role in decision making process? We assume no, as data on patient reported outcomes, like DLQI and HDSS differ from study to study, that no obvious picture of cost-effectiveness is possible. Has quality of life to be considered in decision making process of therapy? Of course, but we suggest, that disease specific quality of life questionnaires have to be created and used for both, effectiveness and cost-effectiveness evaluations over a longer period like 24-36 months. To evaluate not only the severity of hyperhidrosis, but also to measure quality of life in order to justify patient´s expenses for treatment performance and to achieve the best therapeutic outcome will be the main challenge for dermatologists in the future.

Appendix 1. Data Extraction Form

Aspect	Criteria & Code
Content validity Evidence that the domain of an instrument is appropriate relative to its intended use. [11] The conceptual and empirical basis for the items of the instrument. How was the target population involved?	++ Target patients and experts were involved + No patient involvement, other form of content validation given. - Inadequate content validity 0 No information reported.
Construct validity Evidence that supports a proposed interpretation of scores based on theoretical implications associated with the constructs being measured. [11] Does the tool confirm hypothesised differences? [12]	++ At least 75% of results in accordance with hypothesis, based on robust design and method. + Under 75% of results in accordance with specific hypothesis, adequate methods used. - Hypothesis not confirmed or inadequate methods used 0 No information reported
Convergent Validity *Does the tool relate to other tools assessing the same construct? [12]*	++ Correlation > 0.70 + Correlation < 0.70

Aspect	Criteria & Code
	- Correlations not statistically significant. 0 No information reported
Internal Consistency The precision of the scale based on the homogeneity of the scale's items at one point in time (Lohr, 2002).	++ Cronbach alpha 0.70 – 0.95 + Cronbach alpha below 0.70 or above 0.95 - Very low Cronbach alpha, inconsistencies observed. 0 No information reported
Test – retest reliability Does a repeated administration of the tool within a reasonable period of time results in similar results? [12]	++ ICC above 0.70 + ICC below 0.70 - No correlation observed 0 No information reported
Responsiveness The ability of the instrument to detect changes over time OR differences between patients, due to therapy or impact of disease	++ 75% of results showed confirmation of hypothesis, based on an adequate measure. + Less than 75% results confirm hypothesis/conflicting evidence. - Poor or solely based on statistical evidence. 0 No information reported.
Floor & Ceiling Effects Does the tool capture the detail and breadth of real differences among persons?	++ Less than 20% in extremities. - More than 20% in extremities. 0 no information reported.
Interpretability Can qualitative meaning be assigned to the scores? [80]	++ Thresholds provided based on anchor or banding techniques + Distribution based techniques used 0 no information reported.
MCID Has the minimal change relevant to patients been reported?	++ MCID reported. 0 MCID not known.
Respondent Burden Is length and content acceptable to patients?	++ Less than 10 minutes - More than 10 minutes or problems with acceptability 0 no information reported
Structure Evidence in support of the proposed structure or scaling of the instrument	++ Item Response theory confirms proposed structure + Factor analysis confirms proposed structure - Factors analysis and item response theory could does not confirm proposed structure 0 No information provided

References

[1] *Harrisons Innere Medizin.* 2012, Berlin: ABW Wiss. Verl.-Ges.

[2] Brinckmann, W., R. Hampel, and R. Andresen, *Hyperhidrosis Differentialdiagnose und aktuelle Therapie*. 1. Aufl. ed. UNI-MED Science. 2006, Bremen: UNI-MED Verl. 84 S.

[3] Kreyden, O.P. and E.P. Scheidegger, Anatomy of the sweat glands, pharmacology of botulinum toxin, and distinctive syndromes associated with hyperhidrosis. *Clin Dermatol, 2004*. 22(1): p. 40-4.

[4] Sato, K., et al., Biology of sweat glands and their disorders. I. Normal sweat gland function. *J Am Acad Dermatol,* 1989. 20(4): p. 537-63.

[5] Gelbard, C.M., H. Epstein, and A. Hebert, Primary pediatric hyperhidrosis: a review of current treatment options. *Pediatr Dermatol,* 2008. 25(6): p. 591-8.

[6] Lowe, N., et al., The place of botulinum toxin type A in the treatment of focal hyperhidrosis. *Br J Dermatol,* 2004. 151(6): p. 1115-22.

[7] Lowe, N.J., et al., Botulinum toxin type A in the treatment of primary axillary hyperhidrosis: a 52-week multicenter double-blind, randomized, placebo-controlled study of efficacy and safety. *J Am Acad Dermatol,* 2007. 56(4): p. 604-11.

[8] Bechara, F.G., et al., Assessment of quality of life in patients with primary axillary hyperhidrosis before and after suction-curettage. *J Am Acad Dermatol,* 2007. 57(2): p. 207-12.

[9] Hamm, H., et al., Primary focal hyperhidrosis: disease characteristics and functional impairment. *Dermatology,* 2006. 212(4): p. 343-53.

[10] Worle, B., S. Rapprich, and M. Heckmann, Definition and treatment of primary hyperhidrosis. *J Dtsch Dermatol Ges,* 2007. 5(7): p. 625-8.

[11] Aaronson, N., et al., Assessing health status and quality-of-life instruments: attributes and review criteria. *Qual Life Res,* 2002. 11(3): p. 193-205.

[12] Both, H., et al., Critical review of generic and dermatology-specific health-related quality of life instruments. *J Invest Dermatol,* 2007. 127(12): p. 2726-39.

[13] Strutton, D.R., et al., US prevalence of hyperhidrosis and impact on individuals with axillary hyperhidrosis: results from a national survey. *J Am Acad Dermatol*, 2004. 51(2): p. 241-8.

[14] Augustin, M., et al., Prevalence and disease burden of hyperhidrosis in the adult population. *Dermatology,* 2013. 227(1): p. 10-3.

[15] Augustin, M., et al., Prevalence of skin lesions and need for treatment in a cohort of 90 880 workers. *Br J Dermatol,* 2011. 165(4): p. 865-73.

[16] Stander, S., et al., Prevalence of chronic pruritus in Germany: results of a cross-sectional study in a sample working population of 11,730. *Dermatology,* 2010. 221(3): p. 229-35.

[17] Fujimoto, T., K. Kawahara, and H. Yokozeki, Epidemiological study and considerations of primary focal hyperhidrosis in Japan: from questionnaire analysis. *J Dermatol,* 2013. 40(11): p. 886-90.

[18] Westphal, F.L., et al., Prevalence of hyperhidrosis among medical students. *Rev Col Bras Cir,* 2011. 38(6): p. 392-7.

[19] Stefaniak, T., et al., Is subjective hyperhidrosis assessment sufficient enough? prevalence of hyperhidrosis among young Polish adults. *J Dermatol,* 2013. 40(10): p. 819-23.

[20] Chu, D., et al., Incidence and frequency of endoscopic sympathectomy for the treatment of hyperhidrosis palmaris in Taiwan. *Kaohsiung J Med Sci,* 2010. 26(3): p. 123-9.

[21] Felini, R., et al., [Prevalence of hyperhidrosis in the adult population of Blumenau-SC, Brazil]. *An Bras Dermatol,* 2009. 84(4): p. 361-6.

[22] Li, X., et al., Epidemiological survey of primary palmar hyperhidrosis in adolescents. *Chin Med J* (Engl), 2007. 120(24): p. 2215-7.

[23] Tu, Y.R., et al., Epidemiological survey of primary palmar hyperhidrosis in adolescent in Fuzhou of People's Republic of China. *Eur J Cardiothorac Surg,* 2007. 31(4): p. 737-9.

[24] Hoorens, I. and K. Ongenae, Primary focal hyperhidrosis: current treatment options and a step-by-step approach. *J Eur Acad Dermatol Venereol,* 2012. 26(1): p. 1-8.

[25] Perera, E. and R. Sinclair, Hyperhidrosis and bromhidrosis -- a guide to assessment and management. *Aust Fam Physician,* 2013. 42(5): p. 266-9.

[26] Walling, H.W. and B.L. Swick, Treatment options for hyperhidrosis. *Am J Clin Dermatol,* 2011. 12(5): p. 285-95.

[27] Cerfolio, R.J., et al., The Society of Thoracic Surgeons expert consensus for the surgical treatment of hyperhidrosis. *Ann Thorac Surg,* 2011. 91(5): p. 1642-8.

[28] Moreno Balsalobre, R., et al., Guidelines on surgery of the thoracic sympathetic nervous system. *Arch Bronconeumol,* 2011. 47(2): p. 94-102.

[29] Holzle, E., et al., Recommendations for tap water iontophoresis. *J Dtsch Dermatol Ges,* 2010. 8(5): p. 379-83.

[30] Solish, N., et al., A comprehensive approach to the recognition, diagnosis, and severity-based treatment of focal hyperhidrosis: recommendations of the Canadian Hyperhidrosis Advisory Committee. *Dermatol Surg,* 2007. 33(8): p. 908-23.

[31] Blome, C., et al., Dimensions of patient needs in dermatology: subscales of the patient benefit index. *Arch Dermatol Res,* 2011. 303(1): p. 11-7.

[32] Frost, M.H., et al., What is sufficient evidence for the reliability and validity of patient-reported outcome measures? *Value Health,* 2007. 10 Suppl 2: p. S94-S105.

[33] de Campos, J.R., et al., Quality of life, before and after thoracic sympathectomy: report on 378 operated patients. *Ann Thorac Surg,* 2003. 76(3): p. 886-91.

[34] Fayers, P. and D. Machin, Quality of Life The Assessment, *Analysis and Interpretation of Patient-reported Outcomes,* 2013, Wiley: [s.l.].

[35] Teale, C., et al., Development, validity, and reliability of the Hyperhidrosis Impact Questionnaire (HHIQ). *Quality of Life Research,* 2002. 11(7): p. 702-702.

[36] Jonathan, W.K., et al., Validity and reliability of the hyperhidrosis disease severity scale (HDSS)1 1 All authors are employees of Allergan, Inc. *Journal of the American Academy of Dermatology,* 2004. 50(3): p. P51.

[37] Naumann, M.K., et al., Effect of botulinum toxin type A on quality of life measures in patients with excessive axillary sweating: a randomized controlled trial. *British Journal of Dermatology,* 2002. 147(6): p. 1218-1226.

[38] Lowe, N., et al., The place of botulinum toxin type A in the treatment of focal hyperhidrosis, in *Br J Dermatol.* 2004: England. p. 1115-22.

[39] David, R.S., et al., US prevalence of hyperhidrosis and impact on individuals with axillary hyperhidrosis: Results from a national survey. *Journal of the American Academy of Dermatology,* 2004. 51(2): p. 241-248.

[40] Solish, N., et al., Prospective Open-Label Study of Botulinum Toxin Type A in Patients with Axillary Hyperhidrosis: Effects on Functional Impairment and Quality of Life. *Dermatologic Surgery,* 2005. 31(4): p. 405-413.

[41] Solish, N., et al., A comprehensive approach to the recognition, diagnosis, and severity-based treatment of focal hyperhidrosis: recommendations of the Canadian Hyperhidrosis Advisory Committee, in *Dermatol Surg.* 2007: United States. p. 908-23.

[42] Keller, S., et al., Diagnosis of palmar hyperhidrosis via questionnaire without physical examination. *Clinical Autonomic Research,* 2009. 19(3): p. 175-181.

[43] Neumayer, C., et al., Limited endoscopic thoracic sympathetic block for hyperhidrosis of the upper limb: reduction of compensatory sweating by clipping T4. *Surg Endosc,* 2004. 18(1): p. 152-6.

[44] Panhofer, P., et al., Improved quality of life after sympathetic block for upper limb hyperhidrosis. *British Journal of Surgery,* 2006. 93(5): p. 582-586.

[45] Ambrogi, V., et al., Bilateral thoracoscopic T2 to T3 sympathectomy versus botulinum injection in palmar hyperhidrosis, in *Ann Thorac Surg.* 2009: Netherlands. p. 238-45.

[46] de Campos, J., et al., Quality of life, before and after thoracic sympathectomy: Report on 378 operated patients. *Annals of Thoracic Surgery,* 2003. 76(3): p. 886-891.

[47] Augustin, M., et al., Validation of a comprehensive Freiburg Life Quality Assessment (FLQA) core questionnaire and development of a threshold system. *Eur J Dermatol,* 2004. 14(2): p. 107-13.

[48] Finlay, A.Y. and G.K. Khan, Dermatology Life Quality Index (DLQI)—a simple practical measure for routine clinical use. *Clinical and Experimental Dermatology,* 1994. 19(3): p. 210-216.

[49] Basra, M.K.A., et al., The Dermatology Life Quality Index 1994–2007: a comprehensive review of validation data and clinical results. *British Journal of Dermatology,* 2008. 159(5): p. 997-1035.

[50] Kowalski, J., Minimal important difference (MID) of the Dermatology Life Quality Index in patients with axillary and palmar hyperhidrosis. *Journal of the American Academy of Dermatology,* 2007. 56(2): p. AB52.

[51] Chren, M.M., et al., Skindex, a quality-of-life measure for patients with skin disease: reliability, validity, and responsiveness, in *J Invest Dermatol.* 1996: United States. p. 707-13.

[52] de Campos, J., et al., Questionário de qualidade de vida em pacientes com hiperidrose primária. *J Pneumol,* 2003. 29(4): p. 178-81.

[53] Augustin, M., et al., Validation and Clinical Results of the FLQA-d, a Quality of Life Questionnaire for Patients with Chronic Skin Disease. *Dermatology and Psychosomatics / Dermatologie und Psychosomatik,* 2000. 1(1): p. 12-17.

[54] Augustin, M., et al., German Adaptation of the Skindex-29 Questionnaire on Quality of Life in Dermatology: Validation and Clinical Results. *Dermatology,* 2004. 209(1): p. 14-20.

[55] Abeni, D., et al., Further Evidence of the Validity and Reliability of the Skindex-29: An Italian Study on 2,242 Dermatological Outpatients. *Dermatology,* 2002. 204(1): p. 43-49.

[56] Nijsten, T.E.C., et al., Testing and Reducing Skindex-29 Using Rasch Analysis: Skindex-17. *J Invest Dermatol,* 2006. 126(6): p. 1244-1250.

[57] Both, H., et al., Critical Review of Generic and Dermatology-Specific Health-Related Quality of Life Instruments. *J Invest Dermatol,* 2007. 127(12): p. 2726-2739.

[58] Prinsen, C.A.C., et al., Health-Related Quality of Life Assessment in Dermatology: Interpretation of Skindex-29 Scores Using Patient-Based Anchors. *J Invest Dermatol,* 2010. 130(5): p. 1318-1322.

[59] Augustin, M., et al., The patient benefit index: a novel approach in patient-defined outcomes measurement for skin diseases. *Arch Dermatol Res,* 2009. 301(8): p. 561-71.

[60] Augustin, M., et al., Development and validation of a new instrument for the assessment of patient-defined benefit in the treatment of acne, in *J Dtsch Dermatol Ges.* 2008: Germany. p. 113-20.

[61] McDowell, I., *Measuring health : a guide to rating scales and questionnaires.* 3rd ed. 2006, Oxford ; New York: Oxford University Press. xvi, 748 p.

[62] Devins, G.M., et al., The emotional impact of end-stage renal disease: importance of patients' perception of intrusiveness and control. *Int J Psychiatry Med,* 1983. 13(4): p. 327-43.

[63] Bieling, P., et al., Factor Structure of the Illness Intrusiveness Rating Scale in Patients Diagnosed with Anxiety Disorders. *Journal of Psychopathology and Behavioral Assessment,* 2001. 23(4): p. 223-230.

[64] Cinà, C.S. and C.M. Clase, The Illness Intrusiveness Rating Scale: A measure of severity in individuals with hyperhidrosis. *Quality of Life Research,* 1999. 8(8): p. 693-698.

[65] Streiner, D.L. and G.R. Norman, *Health measurement scales a practical guide to their development and use.* 4th ed ed. 2008, Oxford: Oxford Univ. Pr. XVII, 431 S.

[66] Keller, S., Sekons, M, D., A novel scale for assessing quality of life following bilateral endoscopic thoracic sympathectomy for palmer and plantar hyperhidrosis, in *4th International Symposium on Sympathetic Surgery* 2001 Tampere, Finland.

[67] Lewis, V.J. and A.Y. Finlay, A Critical Review of Quality-of-Life Scales for Psoriasis. *Dermatologic Clinics,* 2005. 23(4): p. 707-716.

[68] Dréno, B., Assessing Quality of Life in Patients with Acne Vulgaris: Implications for Treatment. *American Journal of Clinical Dermatology,* 2006. 7(2): p. 99-106.

[69] Cetindag, I.B., et al., Long-term Results and Quality-of-Life Measures in the Management of Hyperhidrosis. *Thoracic Surgery Clinics,* 2008. 18(2): p. 217-222.

[70] Solish, N., Assessing hyperhidrosis disease severity and impact on quality of life. *Cutis,* 2006. 77(Suppl. 5): p. 17-27.

[71] Veenhof, C., et al., Psychometric evaluation of osteoarthritis questionnaires: A systematic review of the literature. *Arthritis Care & Research,* 2006. 55(3): p. 480-492.

[72] Panhofer, P., et al., A survey and validation guide for health-related quality-of-life status in surgical treatment of hyperhidrosis. *European Surgery,* 2005. 37(3): p. 143-152.

[73] Muller, C., et al., Relative bioavailability and pharmacodynamic effects of methantheline compared with atropine in healthy subjects. *Eur J Clin Pharmacol,* 2012. 68(11): p. 1473-81.

[74] Goh, C.L., Aluminum chloride hexahydrate versus palmar hyperhidrosis. Evaporimeter assessment. *Int J Dermatol,* 1990. 29(5): p. 368-70.

[75] Scholes, K.T., et al., Axillary hyperhidrosis treated with alcoholic solution of aluminium chloride hexahydrate. *Br Med J,* 1978. 2(6130): p. 84-5.

[76] Dressler, D. and F. Adib Saberi, Towards a dose optimisation of botulinum toxin therapy for axillary hyperhidrosis: comparison of different Botox((R)) doses. *J Neural Transm,* 2013. 120(11): p. 1565-7.

[77] Moffat, C.E., W.G. Hayes, and I.K. Nyamekye, Durability of botulinum toxin treatment for axillary hyperhidrosis. *Eur J Vasc Endovasc Surg,* 2009. 38(2): p. 188-91.

[78] Lecouflet, M., et al., Duration of efficacy increases with the repetition of botulinum toxin A injections in primary palmar hyperhidrosis: A study of 28 patients. *J Am Acad Dermatol,* 2014. 70(6): p. 1083-7.

[79] Lecouflet, M., et al., Duration of efficacy increases with the repetition of botulinum toxin A injections in primary axillary hyperhidrosis: a study in 83 patients. *J Am Acad Dermatol,* 2013. 69(6): p. 960-4.

[80] Veenhof, C., et al., Psychometric evaluation of osteoarthritis questionnaires: a systematic review of the literature. *Arthritis Rheum,* 2006. 55(3): p. 480-92.

In: Hyperhidrosis
Editor: Janine R. Huddle

ISBN: 978-1-63321-516-0

Chapter VI

Hyperhidrosis: Causes and Treatments

Ana Carolina Urbaczek*[1]*, Camila Tita Nogueira*[2]*,
***Luiz Fernando Takase*[3] *and Patrícia Rodella*[2;4]**
[1]Universidade de São Paulo, São Carlos, SP, Brasil
[2]Universidade Estadual Paulista Júlio de Mesquita Filho, Araraquara, SP, Brasil
[3]Universidade Federal de São Carlos, Sao Carlos, SP, Brasil
[4]Centro Universitário da Fundação Educacional de Barretos, Barretos, SP, Brasil

Abstract

Sweating helps to regulate body temperature by cooling via the evaporation of sweat produced by sweat glands. Hyperhidrosis is a condition characterized by constant and increased production of sweat by sweat glands, and may be local (primary) or generalized (secondary). Primary hyperhidrosis is a constant and excessive sweating disorder, of unknown cause, that occurs mainly in the axilla, palms, soles of feet and craniofacial region, and more than one area may be involved. The secondary form is caused by a latent condition, such as an infection, endocrine or metabolic disorder, neoplasic disease, neurological condition, psychiatric disorder, spinal cord injury and respiratory or cardiovascular problems. Hyperhidrosis is a clinical manifestation that significantly interferes in an individual's life, causing emotional and social problems, a lower quality of life, physical discomfort and increased risk of skin infections. In general treatment is symptomatic, and varies according to the intensity of the disease. In less severe cases it is customary to use creams and antiperspirant deodorants based on aluminium chloride. In intermediate cases the treatment of choice is oxybutynin. Severe cases require invasive modes of therapy, and are more likely in the adult population. The most widely used form of treatment is thoracic sympathectomy, but most patients experience recurrence of the manifestation in another region of the body (compensatory hyperhidrosis or reflex) after surgery, in the absence of full resolution. The application of botulinum toxin is an alternative approach, although sweating is only temporarily reduced. Acupuncture is a form of treatment that has been used with success, because this condition, according to Traditional Chinese Medicine, is caused by a disorder in the metabolism of water, which is responsible for sweat. As acupuncture is based on treating the cause and not just the effect of pathologies, patients who undergo this treatment report a very satisfactory and more efficient outcome compared to those previously cited.

Keywords: Sweating; hyperhidrosis; therapy

Hyperhidrosis is a chronic autonomic disorder characterized by constant and increased sweat production [1], which can be local (primary) or generalized (secondary). [2, 3] Primary hyperhidrosis, usually associated with hyperactivity of the sympathetic nervous system, is characterized by excessive sweating in a localized and symmetrical fashion, especially in the axilla, palms (palmar), soles of the feet (plantar) and craniofacial region. [3-5] In secondary hyperhidrosis, sweating is generalized and may be related to infections, metabolic or endocrine disorders, psychiatric disorders, spinal cord injury or cardio-respiratory problems. [2, 3]

A better understanding of hyperhidrosis, its symptoms, etiology, diagnosis and treatment will require knowledge of sweat gland morphology and the neurophysiological mechanisms related to the regulation of body temperature.

Anatomy and Physiology

The skin contains two types of sweat gland located deep in the dermis or hypodermis: eccrine and apocrine. [6]

Eccrine glands are long, tubular and open at the skin surface. They are found throughout the body, being absent only in the tympanic membrane, lip margins, nipples, labia minora, clitoris and penis. The highest concentrations of these glands are found on the soles of the feet, palms, axilla and face. The sweat secreted by these glands is liquid, transparent, odourless and hypotonic, is composed primarily of water and may contain other substances removed from the blood by the sweat glands, such as sodium chloride, urea, uric acid, proteins and immunoglobulins. [6] The eccrine glands are innervated by cholinergic fibres from the sympathetic nervous system, and are centrally controlled by the hypothalamus. [6]

Apocrine glands are especially large and are associated with hair follicles, discharging their secretion into the hair canal. They appear in large numbers in the axilla, perianal region, areola, scrotum, pubic mound and labia minora (5, 6). The sweat secreted by these glands is thick and yellowish due to its high concentration of proteins and fatty acids; bacteria present on the skin metabolize these substances, producing isovaleric acid and androsterone, which have an unpleasant odour. These glands receive adrenergic innervation, being sensitive to adrenaline (epinephrine) and noradrenaline, and are activated by emotional responses. [6]

Transpiration is the physiological process by which the water in the body is eliminated by sweat secreted by the sweat glands. Heat dissipation is mainly achieved via the evaporation of sweat on the skin surface. [5] Since excessive body temperature can cause denaturation of proteins and enzymes essential for metabolism, mechanisms of heat dissipation are of vital importance in the organism. [6]

Variations in room temperature are monitored by peripheral thermoceptors located mainly in the skin and can lead to possible fluctuation in central body temperature. Changes in blood temperature are detected by thermoceptors located in the hypothalamus, the brain structure associated with the maintenance of homeostasis of the body. An increase in this temperature activates several hypothalamic nuclei responsible for heat dissipation mechanisms, such as tachypnea, cutaneous vasodilatation and sweating. [6]

Fibres from the cerebral cortex that reach the hypothalamus may be responsible for the regulation of transpiration related to emotional responses. [2, 7] Studies suggest that the emotional sweating pathway is independent from the body's thermoregulatory pathway. [8, 9] It is believed that primary hyperhidrosis is caused by disorders in this autonomic pathway that lead to an exacerbated response to emotional stimuli.

Clinical Manifestations

The main clinical manifestation of hyperhidrosis, primary or secondary, is excessive and constant sweating, which significantly interferes with the individual's life, causing emotional, social and physical problems that impair quality of life, daily activities, personal interactions, occupational and leisure activities, often making social interaction difficult and embarrassing and thus leading to patient isolation. [1, 3, 5] This problem should be considered as a serious public health problem since it can propitiate various behavioral disorders such as social phobia, anxiety and depression. [3, 5]

The high level of moisture in the skin caused by excessive sweating can increase the risk of developing skin infections (bacterial or fungal), warts, dermatophytosis and keratolysis. [5, 10, 11]

Axillary hyperhidrosis causes sweat stains on clothing, leading to frequent changes during the day. Excess moisture and increased friction in the region may cause cutaneous maceration. Bromhidrosis, an unpleasant odour arising from the decomposition of sweat and cellular debris from bacteria and fungi, is also commonly reported by patients. [3, 5]

The palmar form causes many problems in activities that require dry hands, such as those involving handling moisture-sensitive materials (such as paper, etc.), delicate work and writing. Everyday actions, like a simple handshake, can be transformed into an embarrassing situation. [3, 5]

Excess moisture on the soles contributes to the development of athlete's foot (chilblains), warts, blisters, infections and bromhidrosis. [5]

Epidemiology

Epidemiological data on the prevalence of primary hyperhidrosis are scarce and insufficient for an accurate estimate, but it is known to affect more than 1 – 2.8% of the world population; however, overall little is known about its existence and its treatment. [3, 12]

Primary hyperhidrosis affects both men and women equally, and its prevalence was found to be highest among people aged 18 – 64 years. The symptoms can start during childhood, adolescence or adulthood for reasons still unknown, but the average age of onset is 25 years. [11, 12] Approximately 82% of patients with primary palmar-plantar hyperhidrosis report an early start in childhood, with the symptoms worsening during adolescence. Axillar hyperhidrosis manifests during adolescence, when the sex glands become more active. [11, 13]

Epidemiologic studies showed that axillary hyperhidrosis affects 51% of patients, the plantar form affects 29% and the facial form affects 20%. [12, 14]

Few studies have reported the natural course of the disease, but the severity of sweating appears to decrease in patients over 50 years. [13, 14]

Causes

Hyperhidrosis occurs mainly due to autonomic nervous system dysfunction, mainly involving the sympathetic pathways. In this pathology the sweat gland shows normal morphology, function and quantities. Although the cause of this disorder is unknown, it might be caused by an abnormal or exaggerated central response to a normal emotional stress. [5] Primary hyperhidrosis is stimulated by emotion and stress, and does not occur during sleep or sedation. Thermoregulation of the body occurs regardless of the level of consciousness, and it is believed that the primary defect in these patients may be a hypothalamic hypersensitivity to an emotional stimulus of the cerebral cortex. [2, 7]

Recent evidence suggests that primary hyperhidrosis has a familial component, indicating a genetic basis for this condition. [13] Approximately 30 – 50% of patients have a family history of hyperhidrosis. [15] A familial variant with autosomal dominant inheritance is now recognized, with some families linked to an abnormality of chromosome14q. [16]

Secondary hyperhidrosis can be drug-induced (i.e. sertraline), toxin-induced (acrylamide) [7], caused by a systemic illness (neoplasms, spinal cord lesions), neurological conditions, psychiatric disorders, respiratory or cardiovascular problems, endocrine or metabolic disorders (hyperthyroidism, menopause or obesity), congenital disorders such as familial dysautonomia (Riley-Day syndrome), by infections or it can be compensatory. [2, 3, 18]

Compensatory hyperhidrosis is a phenomenon in which there is increased sweating in parts of the body unrelated to the location of treatment or in the case of surgery, unrelated to surgery or anatomy. [15] It is often seen in segments below the level of sympathectomy, one of the treatment options. Gustatory hyperhidrosis (usually involving the face) can be familial or occur in association with trauma or other local insults. One epidemiological survey in 2004 estimated that as many as 0.5% of the US population may be suffering from the debilitating effects of hyperhidrosis with major interference in daily activities. [12]

Diagnosis

The first step in evaluation is to differentiate between primary and secondary hyperhidrosis. While primary hyperhidrosis can occur in healthy people, secondary hyperhidrosis usually part of some other underlying condition, such as infective or malignant disease or a hormonal disorder (19). To differentiate these two conditions it is necessary to evaluate the medical history, focusing on the location of excessive sweating, family history, age at onset and the absence of any apparent cause. [14]

The diagnosis of primary hyperhidrosis is basically clinical, not requiring laboratory investigations. [5] The criteria include excessive sweating for at least 6 months without any obvious cause, with a symmetrical pattern of sweating occurring at least once per week.

Since emotional sweating does not occur during sleep or sedation, one of the criteria for diagnosing primary hyperhidrosis is that the patient does not experience sweating during sleep.

The symptom must also impair daily activities have an age of onset younger than 25, cessation of focal sweating during sleep, or a positive family history. [5, 20]

Treatments

If primary diseases such as hyperthyroidism or diabetes are not the etiology, in general the treatment is symptomatic and varies according to the intensity of the hyperhidrosis. Severe cases require invasive therapy, and are more likely in the adult population. Few studies have evaluated the use of treatments in children and adolescents, due to the complications and limitations of each treatment modality, which include: topical therapy with the use of antiperspirants, iontophoresis, botulinum toxin injection, anticholinergic medications, surgical excision and thoracic sympathectomy to interrupt the innervation of sweat glands by the sympathetic nerves. [5, 7, 11]

Topical

Topical agents have been used for axillary, palmoplantar and gustatory hyperhidrosis. [9]

Aluminium salts are the main topical agents for the treatment of hyperhidrosis. Their mechanism of action is attributed to either mechanical obstruction of the eccrine gland duct or to atrophy of the secretory cells (21). Aluminium chloride-based creams and antiperspirant deodorants are effective only in milder cases and the effects last for only 48 h. [9, 14, 22] In more severe cases the treatment of choice is oxybutynin.

The most commonly observed side effects are localized burning, stinging and irritation, probably due to the high salt concentration. [22]

Systemic Treatment

Although systemic treatment is currently used in patients with secondary hyperhidrosis (14), several studies have assess edits effectiveness in primary hyperhidrosis.

The main systemic drugs used to treat primary hyperhidrosis are anticholinergic agents. The inhibition of synaptic acetylcholine interferes with neuroglandular signalling and reduces sweat production and secretion (23). Despite their potential, these drugs have serious limitations. Long-term therapy is required, and the minimal dose for clinical effectiveness causes adverse effects such as dry mouth, blurred vision, urinary retention, constipation and tachycardia. [4, 14, 23]

The administration of glycopyrrolate led to significant improvement in primary hyperhidrosis; however approximately 30% of the patients presented adverse side effects and were excluded from the test. [24, 25]

Escalating doses of oxybutynin over a period of 12 weeks led to significant improvement in symptoms of axillary hyperhidrosis with minimal side effects. [26] Another study from the same laboratory analysed the effectiveness of long-term oxybutynin treatment. The results showed that 82.9% of patients presented significant improvement in axillary hyperhidrosis after a median of 17 months of treatment. [27]

Anxiolytics can also be used to treat primary hyperhidrosis. The mechanism of action of these agents may be related to the reduction in emotional stimuli that trigger hyperhidrosis. [25] However, anxiolytics have serious side effects, such as dependency, lethargy and drowsiness. [7]

Iontophoresis

Electrical treatments for hyperhidrosis became more popular after the development of more effective iontophoresis devices available for home use. [28] This technique consists of introducing ions into the skin by means of a low amperage direct current. One electrode is placed under the area to be treated in a shallow basin filled with tap water; the other electrode is attached under the contra lateral limb. [14, 29] This procedure is primarily used for palmar and plantar hyperhidrosis, since hands and feet are the easiest body parts to submerge in water. Such treatment may reduce sweating enough for daily application of aluminium chloride hexahydrate to be effective. [14]

Iontophoresis also enhances the transdermal delivery of ionized drugs through the skin, which is the main barrier to drug transport. The addition of anticholinergic agents (i.e. glycopyrronium bromide) to the water increases the effectiveness of the treatment. [29]

The mechanism of action of iontophoresis remains unclear, but two theories are currently offered. In the first, iontophoresis is postulated to selectively target areas with high concentrations of electrolytes. In these areas, local electrochemical coagulation of proteins might obstruct the sweat duct. [30] The second theory postulates that the electrical change produced by tap water iontophoresis disrupts eccrine gland secretion. [30]

Although there are no large randomized controlled trials in the literature, iontophoresis can be considered effective for palmoplantar hyperhidrosis (14). Several uncontrolled trials reported an effectiveness of 80 – 100% after treatment. [31, 32]

Iontophoresis is considered a second-line treatment for focal palmoplantar hyperhidrosis, but this treatment has several limitations. Long-term maintenance therapy is generally required, with 30 minutes per treatment site daily for at least 4 days a week. Due to the electrical nature of iontophoresis, the treatment is contraindicated in pregnant women or patients that have a pacemaker. Skin irritation, dryness and peeling are also observed in patients. [14]

Botulinum Toxin

For individuals who do not wish to undergo surgery and its complications, botulinum toxin (Botox) is an alternative. Botulinum toxin has been known to block postganglionic sympathetic cholinergic fibres to sweat glands, temporarily reducing sweat production for 4 – 10 months. Intradermal injections of this agent are considered safe, effective, and well-tolerated alternative to traditional topical, systemic, or surgical approaches. [33]

The injection of botulinum toxins a treatment for axillary hyperhidrosis led to significant improvement in 95% of patients after 1 week and the effect lasted for 7 months. [1, 34] For palmar hyperhidrosis, the treatment was effective in 90% of patients and lasted for 4 – 6 months. [35]

The major limitation of this treatments that the injections are painful and require local anaesthesia [14].

Surgical Therapy

If topical therapy and botulinum toxin injections are unsuccessful, two types of surgery can be indicated: local destruction of sweat glands or endoscopic thoracic sympathectomy.

Local destruction of sweat glands is commonly indicated for axillary hyperhidrosis. It is performed by suction curettage and/or tumescent liposuction techniques. These procedures can decrease sweating in 70 to 90% of patients. The risk of complications is low and compensatory hyperhidrosis does not occur. [36]

The most widely used form of treatment of palmar hyperhidrosis is endoscopic thoracic sympathectomy. In this approach, the sympathetic ganglia are destroyed by excision, clamping, transection or ablation with cautery or laser at the T2 – T3 level, blocking the nerve impulse to the sweat glands. [14, 37]

Surgery is effective at eliminating axillary, palmar and facial hyperhidrosis in 68–100% of cases; postoperative follow-up showed long-lasting improvements. [38, 39]

Despite the efficacy of sympathectomy, not all patients benefit from it, primarily due to the high financial cost, the surgical risks (anaesthetic and infections) and the exclusion criteria for performing this procedure, such as previous thoracic surgery, pleuropulmonary and heart disease, cancer and overweight. [40]

In addition, symptoms recur in 8.2% of patients with palmar hyperhidrosis and in 13.7% of patients with axillar hyperhidrosis.In20–50% of patients, the local excess sweat is controlled, but other parts of the body start to show excessive sweating, usually on the back and thighs. This effect is known as compensatory or reflex hyperhidrosis, and probably represents a thermo-regulatory response of the organism. [11]

Acupuncture

According to Traditional Chinese Medicine (TCM), the formation, distribution and removal of organic liquids (*Jin-Ye*) are dependent on *Qi* activity, and the functional capacity of the organs (*Zang-Fu*) is related to the metabolism of water, including that of the lungs, spleen/pancreas, kidney, bladder and triple heater. A disorder in the metabolism of water and alterations in the formation of the *Jin-Ye*, due to functional impairment of any of the *Zang-Fu* cited, can cause, among other symptoms, excessive sweating and hyperhidrosis. Acupuncture treatment involves stimulating *Yang* and restoring energetic balance in these organs. [41, 42]

Since acupuncture is based on treating the cause and not just the effect of pathologies, the results achieved for primary hyperhidrosis seem effective and apparently without side effects. This suggests that acupuncture can be considered a valid complementary and/or alternative treatment in hyperhidrosis.

Wang and Zhao in 2008 [43] showed that acupuncture produced more efficient results than traditional Western medicine. Their study included 56 patients: the experimental group (n = 30) was treated with acupuncture, using *Huatuojiaji* (EX-B2) points bilaterally; the control group (n = 26) was treated with Western medicine (1mg of estazolam, orally, three times per day). At the end of this study, 96.7% of patients who received acupuncture treatment showed improvement in symptoms; in the control group, only 57.7% of the patients reported any improvement in symptoms.

Another study treated three patients showing symptoms of hyperhidrosis with acupuncture. The following points were used bilaterally: LI4, LI11, LU3, SP6, KI3, KI7, LR3 and *Taiyang*; other points were used unilaterally: GV14, GV20 and *Yintang*. Complementarily auricular acupuncture was administered. At the end of treatment, all patients showed significant improvements in symptoms. [44]

Despite these positive results, new trials using standardized control groups and rigorous experimental protocols are needed to fully understand the mechanisms of action of acupuncture treatment.

Hyperhidrosis can be considered a serious problem since it causes significant deficits in the patient's quality of life. The treatment of primary hyperhidrosis mainly depends on the severity of the condition. Aluminium chloride-based topical agents and iontophoresis can be used in mild and moderate cases. Systemic treatment has several side effects. Intradermal injections of botulinum toxin show good results in severe cases, but are painful and costly. Surgical therapy is considered the last resort for patients with severe hyperhidrosis that do not respond efficiently to other treatments. Acupuncture has shown good prospects as a complementary and/or alternative treatment. Although these treatments greatly benefit the patient's life, new treatments for primary hyperhidrosis should be developed.

References

[1] Naumann M, Lowe NJ. Botulinum toxin type A in treatment of bilateral primary axillary hyperhidrosis: randomised, parallel group, double blind, placebo controlled trial. *BMJ.* 2001;323(7313):596-9.

[2] Schlereth T, Dieterich M, Birklein F. Hyperhidrosis--causes and treatment of enhanced sweating. *Dtsch Arztebl Int.* 2009;106(3):32-7.

[3] Park EJ, Han KR, Choi H, Kim dW, Kim C. An epidemiological study of hyperhidrosis patients visiting the Ajou University Hospital hyperhidrosis center in Korea. *J Korean Med Sci.* 2010;25(5):772-5.

[4] Hashmonai M, Kopelman D, Assalia A. The treatment of primary palmar hyperhidrosis: a review. *Surg Today.* 2000;30(3):211-8.

[5] Bellet JS. Diagnosis and treatment of primary focal hyperhidrosis in children and adolescents. Semin Cutan Med Surg. 2010;29(2):121-6.

[6] Standring S. *Gray's anatomy : the anatomical basis of clinical practice.* 40 ed. Scotland: Churchill Livingstone/Elsevier; 2008. 1576 p.

[7] Thomas I, Brown J, Vafaie J, Schwartz RA. Palmoplantar hyperhidrosis: a therapeutic challenge. *Am Fam Physician.* 2004;69(5):1117-20.

[8] Saadia D, Voustianiouk A, Wang AK, Kaufmann H. Botulinum toxin type A in primary palmar hyperhidrosis: randomized, single-blind, two-dose study. *Neurology.* 2001;57(11):2095-9.

[9] Lakraj AA, Moghimi N, Jabbari B. Hyperhidrosis: anatomy, pathophysiology and treatment with emphasis on the role of botulinum toxins. *Toxins (Basel).* 2013;5(4):821-40.

[10] de Campos JR, Kauffman P, Werebe EeC, Andrade Filho LO, Kusniek S, Wolosker N, et al. Quality of life, before and after thoracic sympathectomy: report on 378 operated patients. *Ann Thorac Surg.* 2003;76(3):886-91.

[11] de Campos JRM, Kauffman P. Simpatectomia torácica por videotoracoscopia para tratamento da hiperidrose primária. *Jornal Brasileiro de Pneumologia.* 2007;33(3):xv-xvii.

[12] Strutton DR, Kowalski JW, Glaser DA, Stang PE. US prevalence of hyperhidrosis and impact on individuals with axillary hyperhidrosis: results from a national survey. *J Am Acad Dermatol.* 2004;51(2):241-8.

[13] Felini R, Demarchi AR, Fistarol ED, Matiello M, Delorenze LM. [Prevalence of hyperhidrosis in the adult population of Blumenau-SC, Brazil]. *An Bras Dermatol.* 2009;84(4):361-6.

[14] Haider A, Solish N. Focal hyperhidrosis: diagnosis and management. *CMAJ.* 2005;172(1):69-75.

[15] Sato K, Kang WH, Saga K, Sato KT. Biology of sweat glands and their disorders. II. Disorders of sweat gland function. *J Am Acad Dermatol.* 1989;20(5 Pt 1):713-26.

[16] Del Sorbo F, Brancati F, De Joanna G, Valente EM, Lauria G, Albanese A. Primary focal hyperhidrosis in a new family not linked to known loci. *Dermatology.* 2011;223(4):335-42.

[17] Bachmann M, Myers JE, Bezuidenhout BN. Acrylamide monomer and peripheral neuropathy in chemical workers. *Am J Ind Med.* 1992;21(2):217-22.

[18] Leung AK, Chan PY, Choi MC. Hyperhidrosis. *Int J Dermatol.* 1999;38(8):561-7.

[19] Böni R. Generalized hyperhidrosis and its systemic treatment. *Curr Probl Dermatol.* 2002;30:44-7.

[20] Hornberger J, Grimes K, Naumann M, Glaser DA, Lowe NJ, Naver H, et al. Recognition, diagnosis, and treatment of primary focal hyperhidrosis. *J Am Acad Dermatol.* 2004;51(2):274-86.

[21] Hölzle E, Kligman AM. Mechanism of antiperspirant action of aluminum salts. Soc Cosm Chem 1979;30:279-95.

[22] Scholes KT, Crow KD, Ellis JP, Harman RR, Saihan EM. Axillary hyperhidrosis treated with alcoholic solution of aluminium chloride hexahydrate. *Br Med J.* 1978;2(6130):84-5.

[23] Connolly M, de Berker D. Management of primary hyperhidrosis: a summary of the different treatment modalities. *Am J Clin Dermatol.* 2003;4(10):681-97.

[24] Bajaj V, Langtry JA. Use of oral glycopyrronium bromide in hyperhidrosis. *Br J Dermatol.* 2007;157(1):118-21.

[25] Walling HW. Systemic therapy for primary hyperhidrosis: a retrospective study of 59 patients treated with glycopyrrolate or clonidine. *J Am Acad Dermatol.* 2012;66(3):387-92.

[26] Wolosker N, de Campos JR, Kauffman P, Neves S, Munia MA, BiscegliJatene F, et al. The use of oxybutynin for treating axillary hyperhidrosis. *Ann Vasc Surg.* 2011;25(8):1057-62.

[27] Wolosker N, Teivelis MP, Krutman M, de Paula RP, Kauffman P, de Campos JR, et al. *Long-term Results of the Use of Oxybutynin for the Treatment of Axillary Hyperhidrosis.* Ann Vasc Surg. 2014.

[28] Levit F. Simple device for treatment of hyperhidrosis by iontophoresis. *Arch Dermatol.* 1968;98(5):505-7.

[29] Chia HY, Tan AS, Chong WS, Tey HL. Efficacy of iontophoresis with glycopyrronium bromide for treatment of primary palmar hyperhidrosis. *J Eur Acad Dermatol Venereol.* 2012;26(9):1167-70.

[30] Sato K, Timm DE, Sato F, Templeton EA, Meletiou DS, Toyomoto T, et al. Generation and transit pathway of H+ is critical for inhibition of palmar sweating by iontophoresis in water. *J Appl Physiol* (1985). 1993;75(5):2258-64.

[31] Hölzle E, Alberti N. Long-term efficacy and side effects of tap water iontophoresis of palmoplantar hyperhidrosis--the usefulness of home therapy. *Dermatologica.* 1987;175(3):126-35.

[32] Reinauer S, Neusser A, Schauf G, Hölzle E. Iontophoresis with alternating current and direct current offset (AC/DC iontophoresis): a new approach for the treatment of hyperhidrosis. *Br J Dermatol.* 1993;129(2):166-9.

[33] Cohen JL, Solish N. Treatment of hyperhidrosis with botulinum toxin. *Facial Plast Surg Clin North Am.* 2003;11(4):493-502.

[34] Heckmann M, Ceballos-Baumann AO, Plewig G, Group HS. Botulinum toxin A for axillary hyperhidrosis (excessive sweating). *N Engl J Med.* 2001;344(7):488-93.

[35] Lowe NJ, Yamauchi PS, Lask GP, Patnaik R, Iyer S. Efficacy and safety of botulinum toxin type a in the treatment of palmar hyperhidrosis: a double-blind, randomized, placebo-controlled study. *Dermatol Surg.* 2002;28(9):822-7.

[36] Rezai K. Suction curettage of the sweat glands--an update. *Dermatol Surg.* 2009;35(7):1126-9.

[37] Cohen Z, Shinar D, Levi I, Mares AJ. Thoracoscopic upper thoracic sympathectomy for primary palmar hyperhidrosis in children and adolescents. *J Pediatr Surg.* 1995;30(3):471-3.

[38] Lin TS, Fang HY. Transthoracic endoscopic sympathectomy in the treatment of palmar hyperhidrosis--with emphasis on perioperative management (1,360 case analyses). *Surg Neurol.* 1999;52(5):453-7.

[39] Doolabh N, Horswell S, Williams M, Huber L, Prince S, Meyer DM, et al. Thoracoscopic sympathectomy for hyperhidrosis: indications and results. *Ann Thorac Surg.* 2004;77(2):410-4; discussion 4.

[40] Munia MA, Wolosker N, Kauffman P, de Campos JR, Puech-Leão P. A randomized trial of T3-T4 versus T4 sympathectomy for isolated axillary hyperhidrosis. *J Vasc Surg.* 2007;45(1):130-3.

[41] Urbaczek AC, Severo NF, Rodella P, da Costa PI. Tratamiento de la hiperhidrosis palmar primaria por acupuntura. A propósito de un caso. *Rev Int Acupuntura.* 2013;7(3):85-6.

[42] Maciocia G. *Diagnóstico na Medicina Chinesa - Um Guia Geral.* 1 ed: Roca; 2005.

[43] Wang WZ, Zhao L. Acupuncture treatment for spontaneous polyhidrosis. *J Tradit Chin Med.* 2008;28(4):262-3.

[44] Cayir Y, Engin Y. Acupuncture for primary hyperhidrosis: case series. *Acupunct Med.* 2013;31(3):325-6.

In: Hyperhidrosis
Editor: Janine R. Huddle
ISBN: 978-1-63321-516-0

Chapter VII

Surgical Options for the Treatment of Primary Palmar Hyperhidrosis: Consensus and Controversies

Moshe Hashmonai, M.D., F.A.C.S.*
Technion – Israel Institute of Technology,
Faculty of Medicine (Retired)

Abstract

Primary palmar hyperhidrosis (PPHH) is a highly disturbing pathology affecting 0.15-0.25% of the young population, ensuing severe functional and social handicaps. For decades, the second thoracic ganglion (T2) was considered to be responsible for palmar perspiration and its resection was accepted as the golden standard for the surgical treatment of PPHH. However, sympathetic ablation bears several sequels, compensatory hyperhidrosis (CHH) being the gravest and most commonly observed. It consists in increased perspiration of a part of the body unaffected by the sympathetic ablation, and may attain devastating proportions. The mechanism of CCH is complex, enigmatic and obscure. To reduce its magnitude, two major approached were suggested: (a)

* E-mail address: hasmonai@inter.net.il

modification of the surgical procedure by clipping or transecting the sympathetic chain instead of resecting the ganglion, and/or lowering the level of the procedure from T2 to T3-T4; and (b) reversal procedures: unclipping or reconstructing the continuity of the sympathetic chain by nerve grafting. The actual consensus is that appropriate sympathetic ablation is the only treatment which may cure PPHH. All methods of performing the procedure are still debated as are the proposed approaches to reduce CHH. The methods by which results are evaluated are also controversial. QoL is examined by questionnaires, several types of which have been proposed. Comparing QoL before and after surgical sympathetic ablation is usually the method of evaluating results in use. However, this is a subjective method and no comparison of results of different studies is possible. Furthermore, to learn the pathophysiological aspects of a surgical procedure, metrical assessment of results is required. The aim of the present report is to review the literature and present the State of the Art concerning the surgical treatment of PPHH.

Introduction

Hyperhidrosis is a pathological condition of excessive secretion of the eccrine sweat glands in amounts greater than required for physiological needs. [1] It may be secondary to a variety of medical disorders [2] or it may be primary, of unknown etiology. Primary palmar hyperhidrosis (PPHH) affects primarily young persons. Epidemiological data are scant. The study of a young population in Israel showed that 0.6-1.0% complained of excessive sweating of varying degree and anatomical distribution. [3] However, only a quarter of those affected had severe palmar sweating, which represents an incidence of 0.15-0.25% of the population. [3] PPHH may generate severe social, emotional and occupational handicaps at an early age. A multitude of therapeutic modalities have been proposed for the treatment of PPHH. [4, 5] The only treatment which may abolish PPHH is the appropriate sympathetic ablation. The reasons for which the remaining modalities are in use are the sequels of sympathetic surgery which may attain devastating proportions. [6] The purpose of the present review is to summarize the consensus concerning the treatment of PPHH by sympathetic ablation and to define the items in controversy.

Historical Note

In 1852, the physiologist Claude Bernard performed the first sympathetic ablation by severing the sympathetic nerve in a rabbit's neck. [7] His hypothesis was that the consequence would be cooling of the limb, yet he observed and recorded the opposite effect. This experiment was the physiological basis for one of the major indications for sympathetic surgery. Yet the first clinical surgical sympathectomy, performed by Alexander in 1896 [8], was for a different and long since obsolete indication – epilepsy. The first to exploit Claude Bernard's observation was Jaboulay who in 1899 performed a sympathetic ablation by perivascular stripping of the femoral artery in a man afflicted with trophic lesions of the foot. [9] The first sympathetic ablation for the treatment of hyperhidrosis was performed by Kotzareff [10] in 1920. Since this time, the treatment of palmar hyperhidrosis by sympathectomy was rapidly established.

In the first decades of the 20th century, four major approaches to the cervical and upper thoracic sympathetic chain were developed.

Posterior Approach Adson [11] developed the posterior approach, further modified by White et al., [12] and by Smithwick. [13] This approach allows both unilateral and one stage bilateral sympathetic ablation. It is based on preganglionic resection of the white afferent rami and furthermore, it permits resection of the root ganglia and the sympathetic ganglia. [13, 14]

Anterior Transthoracic Approach First suggested by Goetz and Marr [15] in 1942 and later adopted by Palumbo [16], this approach involves a limited anterior thoracotomy.

Axillary Transthoracic Approach This approach was devised by Schultze and Goetz [17] and described and published by Atkins [18] in 1949. It also involves a limited thoracotomy, but the incision is concealed in the axilla.

Supraclavicular Approach Telford described this procedure in 1935. [19] It allows the approach of the stellate and upper thoracic ganglia without penetrating the pleural cavity.

The anterior and posterior approaches were the least popular. The former involves penetrating the pleural cavity and leaves a rather visible scar. The latter, which requires rib section/resection, is the most traumatic. In the era of open surgery, the most popular approaches were the peraxillary and the supraclavicular. The former is easy, but requires penetrating the pleural cavity. Furthermore, although feasible, bilateral surgery was usually performed as a two stage procedure. The supraclavicular approach is technically the most demanding, but recovery is rapid and both sides are easily operated as a one stage procedure.

The first endoscopic approach to the sympathetic chain was published by Hughes [20] in 1942. The only surgeons to widely use an endoscopic approach in the following decades were Kux E [21] and Kux M [22]. Yet, it was only with the advent of endoscopic surgery in the eighties, that the minimal invasive approaches gained popularity, totally supplanting the open techniques which became obsolete. Yet, cases may be met [23], when the endoscopic approach is not feasible and the surgeon should be capable to perform upper sympathetic ablation by one of the open techniques.

Non Surgical Treatments vs. Surgery

A plethora of therapies have been reported and are still been used. [4, 5, 24-27] They include noninvasive treatments with central effect (hypnosis, psychotherapy, biofeedback, tranquilizing drugs), and treatments with peripheral effect (topical external ointments: antiperspirants, astringents, anticholinergics; iontophoresis; local radiation; cryotherapy). However, none of these treatments may assure permanent cure. Invasive nonsurgical treatments include locally injected drugs (botulinum) and percutaneous radiofrequency ablation or CT guided phenol block. Botulinum injections offer a temporary relief, require repeated treatments, and are not devoid of complications and side effects. [28] Although in a series of 110 patients radiofrequency upper thoracic ablation produced complete or largely interrupted sympathetic activity in 96% at two years and 91% at three years [29], the method did not gain popularity. Percutaneous sympathetic ablation was successfully achieved with CT guided phenol blocks, but contrary to the surgical procedures, bear a high recurrence rate: Adler et al., [30] reported 41.6% failures at two years follow-up. Appropriate surgical ablation is the only means to secure permanent abolition of palmar sweating. In a review of the literature, in 528 patients who underwent resection of the T2-T3 ganglia in 1020 limbs, the immediate success rate was 99.76% and there were no recurrences. [31] If results are so good, why did not this method been adopted exclusively? The reason is the occurrence and severity of complications and sequels which vary with the various methods of ablation.

The Level of the Required Sympathetic Ablation

The anatomy of the upper thoracic sympathetic system and the sympathetic innervation of the upper limb are complex. [32] The sympathetic nerve fibers emerge from the spinal cord through the ventral roots of the corresponding spinal nerves and pass into the spinal nerve trunks and the commencement of their ventral rami where they leave by communicating braches, the *white rami communicantes*, to join either the sympathetic ganglia on the sympathetic trunk or the interganglionic portions of the trunks. Having reached the sympathetic trunk, the fibers may either synapse with neurons of the corresponding ganglion, or may proceed through the ganglion, either cranially or caudally, to end in a similar way in ganglia at different levels. Thus, although there is no sympathetic outflow from the cervical spinal cord, the cervical ganglia receive their sympathetic innervation via ascending nerve fibers. From the sympathetic ganglia, post ganglionic fibers, the *grey rami communicantes*, emerge to join the corresponding spinal nerves. The grey rami emerging from the sympathetic ganglia join the corresponding spinal nerves and through their ventral and dorsal branches are distributed to the target organs. From the cervical ganglia and mainly from the lower ganglion (part of the stellate ganglion), grey rami join the brachial plexus. [32] The sympathetic input to the upper limb is thus supplied via the brachial plexus and distal nerves from which nerve fibers are contributed to the arterial network of the limb. Some fibers may pass directly to blood vessels in the neighborhood of the sympathetic trunk and may be carried along these vessels and their branches towards their peripheral distribution. The second thoracic ganglion is considered to be the main direct contributor of post ganglionic fibers to the upper limb. [32] Occasionally, synapsing of preganglionic fibers to neurons from which post ganglionic fibers originate occurs in intermediate or accessory ganglia situated proximal to the sympathetic trunk. Some efferent fibers may thus bypass the sympathetic trunk and ganglia. [33] Kuntz at al [34] demonstrated that the sympathetic outflow from the spinal cord to the upper limb is from the first, second and third thoracic segments. This statement was subsequently contested by Hyndman and Wolkin [35] who, based on clinical observations, pertained that in humans, the first thoracic nerve root does not contain sympathetic fibers. In a study of root nerve stimulation in humans [36], it was found that almost invariably the second thoracic segment (T2) was the uppermost contributor to the sympathetic innervation to the upper limb, the lower one being the fifth, although rarely, sympathetic outflow to the hand was found to stem from segments as low as the eight.

In the past, excision of the stellate ganglion (the fusion of the lower sympathetic ganglion with the first thoracic ganglion) together with the second thoracic ganglion was considered to be the standard procedure to obtain sympathetic denervation of the upper limb. [11-13, 34, 35] Additional resection of the corresponding nerve roots with the possible ablation of accessory ganglia if present was considered to secure complete sympathetic denervation of the limb. [33] Lemmens has shown that when relapses occurred following stellate and second thoracic ganglion excision, additional resection of the ventral roots of the second and third spinal nerves were beneficial. [14] However, this type of sympathetic ablation involves sympathetic denervation of the face and head and, most important, it induces Horner's syndrome. To avoid this complication, a more limited approach was adopted. Sympathetic innervation of the pupil was found to stem from the first thoracic segment. [36] Preserving the stellate ganglion, which includes the first thoracic ganglion, secures the sympathetic innervation of the pupil and avoids Horner's syndrome. Telford [19] transected the sympathetic chain below the third ganglion as well as the white rami of the third and second ganglion. Smithwick [37] added transection of the grey rami of these ganglia, raised the third ganglion, rotated it upwards and fixed it in this position to the intercostal muscle. Subsequently, several authors stressed the importance of the second thoracic ganglion in the sympathetic supply of the upper limb and considered this procedure sufficient to obtain palmar anhidrosis. [15, 38-42] Nevertheless, many surgeons ablated the third ganglion and, not infrequently, the first as well. [3, 43-51]

Until the advent of endoscopic surgery, a consensus was thus achieved, the second thoracic ganglion being the target organ for ablation in order to obtain palmar anhidrosis. This consensus was challenged by the advent of thoracoscopy. Several reasons were responsible for this change in concept, the main being the hypothesis that compensatory hyperhidrosis (CHH) is reduced by lowering the level of the sympathetic ablation. [52] CHH is a sequel of sympathetic ablation, it consists in the increase of sweating in areas of the body unaffected by the sympathetic procedure, and in a small percentage of cases may attain devastating proportions. [53] A plethora of articles have been published, each advocating a different level and/or extend of ablation, claiming that, based on the authors' data, the suggested level is the best. Suffice is to state, that there are also opposite publications, claiming that the amount of CHH is not affected by lowering the level of ablation. [53] Limiting the extend of ablation was also considered beneficial to reduce CHH. [54] However, comparing ablation of T2 only versus T2-T3 in two different studies showed no difference in the resulting CHH. [53, 55] In a review of the literature, compilation of results did not support the claim that lowering the level of ablation reduced the severity of CHH. [56] Nevertheless, the balance of reducing the surgical procedure versus decreasing the gravity of CHH remains a major domain of controversy, each surgeon advocating his own point of view. Although insufficiently supported, the impression is that lowering the level does reduce the amount and/or severity of CHH, but increases the percentage of recurrences. [57] Based on this belief, two articles have been published. Balsalobre et al., [58] published "guidelines" for surgery of the thoracic sympathetic system. These guidelines are, however, based on a very restricted review of the literature, which represents a major drawback of their recommendations. Cerfolio et al., [59] published an "expert consensus" on the matter. It is based only on the 12 clinical trials retrieved for the years 1991-2009. Their conclusion is that for palmar hyperhidrosis, interruption of the sympathetic trunk above the third rib is the procedure of choice. The authors are certainly leading figures in the field. However, this consensus has two biases. Two of the 12 trials are redundant publications and the implications are clear. [60] Secondly, its recommendation is based on rib level ablation, not anatomical level of the trunk and the location of the second thoracic ganglion (G2) is known to be inconstantly located in the second intercostal space. Satyapal et al., [61] found the G2 to be located in the second intercostal space in about 90% of cases. Contrary to their study, Chung et al., [62], found the ganglion to be located in this location in only 50% of the cadavers they studied and in about a quarter of the cases, its location was on the upper border of the third rib or over this rib. Furthermore, rib count is often erroneous. Satyapal et al., [61] claimed that the first rib is not visible at thoracoscopy. The same claim is occasionally made in various reports. On the other hand, Wong [63] was able see the first rib in half of cadaveric cases studied and this rib was palpable in the remaining. These controversial reports clarify and underline the importance to visualize the sympathetic trunk and ganglia during sympathetic surgery, and perform the ablation according to anatomical ganglionic identification, not by rib count. Indeed, failure of sympathetic ablation has been attributed to erroneous rib count. [64] If rib count is used, it should be confirmed during surgery by a chest radiograph.

Another change of approach is the method of ablation. Resection and extirpation of the ganglia was the method of choice. In the attempt to reduce and/or attenuate the degree of CHH, many variations of the method of ablation were published. In a review article on sympathetic ablation for palmar hyperhidrosis [56], the authors identified 42 different methods of ablation. Recently two more techniques were added: a transumbilical approach [65] and the use of robot. [66] In an animal study [67], the investigator managed to perform bilateral sympathectomy via the esophagus. No one has attempted so far to use this approach on humans! Apparently, feasibility and desirability are not synonyms.

It seems that the actual trend in thoracoscopic sympathectomy for palmar hyperhidrosis is to lower the level of ablation to T3 and to restrict the extend of ablation. However, in judging the appropriate level and method of sympathetic ablation for palmar hyperhidrosis, the surgeon must base his decision on anatomy, namely, the sympathetic pathways to the palms. In reviewing the literature, it appears that one incentive for the idea of lowering the level of ablation for palmar hyperhidrosis was the "Lin-Telaranta" classification. [68] These authors presented a complex description of neurological sympathetic pathways from the brain, down to the target organs (face, axilla, palms) and back. Based on this "neuroanatomy", they suggested that to alleviate palmar hyperhidrosis, the appropriate level for sympathetic ablation was G4 (clamping the trunk at R4 and R5). However, their "neuroanatomical" description was not confirmed by any anatomical study and, apparently, cannot be confirmed by in vivo studies in humans. It remains a mere hypothesis. Not presenting their view as such undermines the validity of their guidelines. Furthermore, sympathetic ablation for hyperhidrosis is a peripheral procedure and all that matters are the peripheral sympathetic pathways. According to the study of the sympathetic pathways exciting the spine (in vivo in humans) [36], transecting the sympathetic trunk above the G2, transecting the gray rami of G2 and ablating any bypassing fibers like the nerve of Kuntz, will secure complete palmar sympathetic ablation. Any deviation from this procedure, like lowering the level of ablation to G3, although it may reduce and/or attenuate CHH, exposes the patient to incomplete sympathectomy of the hand with all its implications. This statement does not condemn lowering the level of sympathetic ablation for palmar hyperhidrosis, but in obtaining the informed consent, the patient must be supplied with this information.

The Methods of Sympathetic Ablation – Principles

With the advent of endoscopic surgery, the thoracoscopic approach to the sympathetic chain supplanted the four open surgical approaches which became obsolete. Thoracoscopy simplified the operative procedure. The thoracic cavities are approached by very small incisions (one to three), and the ganglia may be cauterized instead of being dissected and excised. [69, 70] Thus, the operation was shortened and less skill demanding. [71] Although the thoracic cavity is invaded on both sides, recovery in the postoperative period became much easier and the operation has been even performed under sedation and local anesthesia on outpatient basis. [72] In an early review of nearly 900 cases, irrespective of the technique, the common denominator of thoracoscopies was simplicity, expedience, minimal surgical trauma, few complications, and low cost compared to standard methods of open surgery. [73] There is no consensus about the optimal method of thoracoscopic sympathetic ablation. The three basic techniques of sympathetic ablation are excision with extirpation, transection, and in situ ablation –thermodestruction. Extirpation secures ablation and allows histological confirmation. Transection may be performed by diathermy, scissors or clipping. The first two methods do not exclude the possibility of nerve regeneration, which has been proven in experimental studies in cats [74, 75] and shown to develop in humans after cardiac transplant. [76] Clipping produces a permanent block of nerve conduction. It has been preferred by surgeons because of the possible reversal procedure by unclipping, should unbearable CHH develop. Another advantage of clipping is that it allows subsequent determination of the ablation level by chest radiography. The drawbacks of thermoablation are the ablated structure being left in situ which may possibly serve as a pathway for nerve regeneration, and the dissipation of heath which may ablate unintended levels and structures.

Recurrence of perspiration was related to either incomplete ablation or to nerve regeneration (sprouting). [77-79] Incomplete ablation may be due to existing sympathetic pathways or to incomplete interruption of the targeted sympathetic ablation. [80] It has been shown that surgical transection of the majority of sympathetic pathways to a target organ achieves complete functional sympathetic block, but after a certain period, the remaining small percentage of unaffected sympathetic pathways may compensate for the block and renovate its sympathetic activity. [78] For the palm, although T2 resection initially achieves complete anhidrosis, the bypassing pathways via the nerve of Kuntz and T3, may allow recurrent perspiration at a latter period of time. [78] A clinical example are the results obtained by the same group of surgeons, comparing their open procedures in which T2-T3 resection was performed [51] to their endoscopic procedures in which, in addition to the T2-T3 resection, the nerve of Kuntz and possible similar fibers were transected as well. [81] In the open group, 4.1% of recurrences were observed compared to 0% for the endoscopic procedures.

Appropriate resympathectomy secures palmar sympathetic denervation. Before reoperation, the exact initial surgical procedure should be assessed. This will allow choosing correctly the required additional ablation. Several studies have reported excellent results of resympathectomy. [80, 82, 83]

Compensatory Hyperhidrosis

Compensatory hyperhidrosis (CHH) is the increase of perspiration after sympathetic denervation for hyperhidrosis occurring in a sympathetically non denervated area of the body. Probably, the earliest observation of this phenomenon was done by Ross [84], who used the term "compensatory hyperhidrosis". Shelley and Florence [85], considered it to be a thermoregulatory phenomenon, namely that the total amount of body perspiration remains unchanged by sympathectomy, whereas the sweating area is decreased. Shoenfeld et al., [86], in a human study found no statistical difference in the total amount of body perspiration before and after "cervical" sympathetic ablation (actually, the procedure was an upper dorsal sympathectomy). The concept of compensation, however, does not explain some clinical observations. CHH does not develop in all sympathicomized patients [87]; it does not necessarily present immediately but may appear as late as six months postoperatively [88]; the degree of CHH is variable [81]; and it may be alleviated or disappear spontaneously. [85, 89] Finally, it has been shown that drying the area of CHH by Botox injections did not incite CHH in a new area. [90] The compensatory mechanism of CHH has been recently challenged by a human study as well. In this study, the total amount of body perspiration in response to a heath stimulus was measured before and after sympathectomy (T2-T3 resection). [91] The total body amount of perspiration before and after surgery was not identical, and there was no correlation between the degree of alteration and the development of CHH. The term "compensatory hyperhidrosis" appears to be a misnomer. The term "reflex sweating" has been proposed as a replacement. However, the phenomenon is not a reflex (the neurological effect of a neurological stimulus) and there is no point to replace a long used misnomer by a new misnomer.

CHH occurs by whichever approach sympathetic ablation is performed. To treat CHH had it occurred, three methods have been proposed: botulinum injections, unclipping to reverse the ablation, and nerve reconstruction.

Botox injections of the area of increased perspiration has been used successfully. [90] Apparently, abolition of CHH did not increase the amount of sweating in another, new area. The major drawback of this method is that the effect of Botox is temporary and in this study [90], the duration of the Botox effect was found to last 2-8 months.

Clipping of nerves obstructs neural transmission. [92] It has been measured that the bursting pressure (the pressure required to open and move a clip) of metal clips varied between 737 and 854 mmHg. [93] Under such pressure, the tissue enclosed within the clip loses its blood supply and invariably must undergo ischemic necrosis. Consequently, clips may be used to discontinue neural transmission through the clipped nerve. Accordingly, on pathophysiological basis, clipping is equivalent to cutting of the nerve and this has been proven in a clinical comparative study. [94] For sympathetic ablation, the advantage of clipping versus transection by diathermy is that no heath is dissipated and no adjacent structures are affected by the procedure. Discordance begins when unclipping is suggested for reversal of sympathetic ablation. Lin et al., [95], reported a series of 326 patients with PPHH who underwent a T2 sympathetic block by clipping. They claimed that, because of severe CHH in 5 patients, clips were removed (pulled out, because only one port was used), 9 to 59 days after the clipping procedure. In four patients, recovery of CHH began 6 to 40 days later. This publication stimulated the use of clipping (and unclipping for reversal). Several publications reported a variable percentage of success due to unclipping. [96-97] The improvement of CHH after clip removal was based on a subjective basis (use of a visual scale, patient's evaluation). No objective measurements were reported. Until recently, the histology of the clipped tissue at different dates post unclipping, or the histology of the sympathetic pathways proximal and distal to the clipped area, has not been examined. Naturally, such tests cannot be performed in humans but are feasible in animals. Recently, two such studies have been published. Loscertales et al., [98] examined the pathology of the sympathetic trunk within and adjacent to the clip at the time of removal, up to 30 days after clipping; and up to 20 days after unclipping. No amyelinated fibers were found after unclipping and the sparse myelinated fibers never crossed the clipped area. Their conclusion was that clipping was not a reversible procedure. To the same conclusion came the other group of investigators [99], who performed a double clipping on the sympathetic trunk of rabbits for 48 hours. In one group, the section of the trunk containing the clipped area was excised whereas in the second group the same segment was excised 45 days after unclipping. Severe degeneration of the sympathetic trunk and ganglion was observed 48 hours after clipping. Forty five days after unclipping, instead of regeneration progressive axonal degeneration was observed. These two short term studies cast a serious doubt about reversibily of sympathetic ablation by unclipping. To obtain a completely decisive conclusion, long-term animal studies are required. Yet, in view of these two studies, how can we analyze the published results of unclipping in humans? Various biases are common to all reports: the evaluation is subjective – no objective measurement of perspiration was ever made in these patients; we do not know the exact mechanism of CHH and therefore cannot evaluate whether unclipping has a certain degree a placebo effect; CHH may alleviate spontaneously and no comparative group of unclipped patients was examined parallel to the clipped group. Therefore, concerning human studies, an objective detailed quantitative documentation is needed. Until such data are provided, when asked for an informed consent, patients who are submitted to unclipping must be advised about the limited and empirical knowledge on the subject. The validity of unclipping remains for now controversial.

The third possibility to reverse the sympathetic ablation was proposed by Telaranta [100], who used a nerve graft to bridge the gap in the sympathetic trunk resulting from the previous sympathectomy. The technical feasibility of such grafting has been proven and found to be successful in an animal model. [101] Based on Telaranta's publication, a few groups of surgeons have performed and published results of nerve graft reconstructions. Haam et al. [102] performed nerve reconstruction in 19 patients of whom, CHH was improved in nine, but markedly improved only in three. However, evaluation of results is difficult because the series includes several kinds of sympathetic ablations performed for three indications. Furthermore, they did not report to what extend the original HH recurred. Wong et al., [103], reported a single case who had an initial T2-T4 sympathetic trunk resection in whom, six months later, a 7 cm nerve graft was used to bridge the resulting gap in the chain. Their patient reported improved trunkal CHH after a month and some degree of recurrent original sweating.

Nerve regeneration is a complicated process, regulated and influenced by local and general factors that are not all fully known. Clinically, regeneration is faster in younger people, has better chances of success the earlier repair is performed, crush injuries fare better than transected lesions, and finally, the distance between the site of injury and the target organ is of paramount importance as axons that need to travel only a short distance to reach their target tissue are more likely to reconnect. [104] Technique of repair and, in case a graft is required because of a gap in the nerve continuity resulting from injury, the type and length of the graft are additional factors, the longer the graft, the longer it takes for axons to cross it. [105] The pace of regeneration is very slow [about 1 mm/d [106]].

Peripheral nerve regeneration has been extensively studied. Regeneration and repair of the sympathetic system has been only scantly investigated. Sympathetic re-innervation has been observed in some transplanted organs [heart [107], intestine [108], veins [109], and sweat glands [110], but not kidneys [111]]. Reconstruction by nerve grafting of postganglionic sympathetic pathways to the prostate has been successful. [112] Re-innervation of ganglionic neurons in the sympathetic chain has also been successfully performed in a study on guinea pigs. [113] The nerve transplant in this experiment was another section of the sympathetic chain and included a ganglion. Axons from the afferent part of the chain were found to sprout and re-synapse with neurons in the transplanted ganglion. In the operation proposed by Telaranta, no sympathetic ganglia are implanted. Therefore, the postganglionic sympathetic innervation to the palms, sprouting from the ablated ganglia cannot be regenerated. Nor can the sympathetic input of ablated pre-ganglionic pathways (white rami communicantes) to the ablated ganglia be regenerated by peripheral nerve grafting to the chain. Thus, it cannot be expected that re-innervation by peripheral nerve grafting performed to bridge the gap resulting from the sympathetic ablation for palmar hyperhidrosis will return the state of perspiration of the palms to pre-sympathectomy levels. If the degree of CHH depends on the amount of ablated postganglionic fibers to the palms, sympathetic reconstruction cannot possibly completely reverse CHH. Furthermore, whatever degree of success is achieved, this may be expected only after a long period of time following reconstruction. The pace of sympathetic axonal growth, although it may be different than that of motor-sensory axons, is very slow as well. Results of the animal study in which a peripheral nerve graft was used [112] were evaluated after 20 months. Accordingly, reported high grade successes, shortly after reconstruction, are baffling. One can, therefore, expect only partial success from nerve reconstruction, and that on long-term follow-up. These possibilities and limitations of reversal operations by nerve grafting must be understood and taken under consideration when such an operation is proposed to a patient.

Unilateral Hyperhidrosis: Is There Contralateral Sympathetic Input?

Unilateral focal hyperhidrosis is a very rare condition. In most of the cases, the affected regions are the head and the forearm. [114] Primary unilateral palmar hyperhidrosis is even rarer. Kopelman et al., [115] published two such cases with dripping right palms. T2-T3 sympathectomy was performed on the affected side of both patients and palmar anhidrosis was obtained. In less than one month, the same degree of hyperhidrosis developed on the other side in both cases. The second side was operated as well in the two patients. The puzzling event in these two cases was that hyperhidrosis recurred on the first operated side less than one month following the second sympathectomy. The method of ablation in all operations was unilateral excision of the T2-T3 ganglia, confirmed by pathology as well as by chest radiographs to assess the level of the procedure. This type of ablation results almost invariable in permanent sympathetic denervation of the palms. [5] The sudden recurrence of palmar hyperhidrosis in these two cases is baffling and unexplained by the known anatomy and physiology of the sympathetic system. Is there an additional factor that may stimulate sweating besides the sympathetic system? Is there a possible sympathetic crossover input? This possibility is supported by another case of RSD pain in one upper limb which could be only temporary relieved by ipsilateral sympathetic blocks. Substantial improvement was achieved only after a contralateral stellate ganglion block was performed. [116] An open question remains: what should be done in a case of unilateral palmar hyperhidrosis? Should only the ipsilateral side be operated exposing the patient to the possibility of subsequent contralateral side hyperhidrosis, or should a bilateral sympathectomy be performed straightforward, exposing the patient to the possibility to develop a more severe CHH? The literature supplies no answer. The subject is enigmatic and remains totally unexplained.

Evaluation of Results - Methods (Patient's Satisfaction vs. Metrics)

Improved quality of life (QoL) is the aim of sympathetic ablation for PPHH. The question is how to assess the improvement. Several questionnaires have been developed for that purpose. [117-121] These kinds of instruments have several drawbacks. They are subjective, relying on the patient. The same results may be evaluated variously by different patients. The satisfaction also depends on the preoperative state of the patient: the worse his preoperative QoL, the better his postoperative evaluation of QoL will be, even if PPHH is not relieved completely. [122-123] However, to estimate the patho-physiological change, objective evaluation is required and provided by metrics. If an estimation of improvement in CHH is to be obtained by a certain procedure, the volume of sweat from a surface unit must be measured before and after the treatment. Several methods have been used: sudometry /gravimetry (transepidermal water loss) [124], evaporimetry (humidity and temperature) [125], skin resistance (conductance) [126], electrical measurement of sweat activity [127], ventilated capsule technique (128), and weight loss (for total body amount of perspiration). [91]

Are metrics superior to subjective evaluation by the patient in assessing sweating? A study considered both methods to be equivalent. [129] However, for scientific purposes quantitative measurements are the only valid method. [130] The benefits of such approach to collecting and presenting data are numerous: objective evaluation, anatomical information, pathophysiological information, precise comparison of data from multiple studies, and the possibility to compile results from such studies.

Conclusion

Until better understanding of the etiological mechanism of primary hyperhidrosis is obtained, the only permanent solution to PPHH is by appropriate sympathetic ablation. The major concern in sympathetic ablation is the sequel of CHH. Further studies are required to understand the mechanism of CHH. Although there is no consensus, it appears that lowering the level of sympathetic ablation and limiting its extend reduces CHH, but the amount of achieved palmar anhidrosis is reduced as well and the percentage of recurrences of PHH is increased. Better and long-term studies are required to evaluate the potentials of unclipping and of nerve graft reconstruction, should reversal of the sympathetic ablation be sought because of severe CHH. Anatomical knowledge of the sympathetic input to the hand is crucial in understanding the merits and pitfalls of sympathetic surgery for PPHH.

References

[1] Sato K, Kang WH, Saga K, Sato KT. Biology of the sweat glands and their disorders II. Disorders of sweat gland function. *J. Am. Acad. Dermatol.* 1989; 20:713-726.

[2] Sato K. Hyperhidrosis. *JAMA* 1991; 265:651.

[3] Adar R, Kurtchin A, Zweig A, Mozes M. Palmar hyperhidrosis and its surgical treatment: a report of 100 cases. *Ann. Surg*. 1977; 186:34-41.

[4] Connoly M, de Berker D. Management of primary hyperhidrosis. A summary of the different treatment modalities. *Am. J. Clin. Dermatol.* 2003; 4:681-697.

[5] Hashmonai M, Kopelman D, Assalia A. The treatment of primary palmar hyperhidrosis: a review. *Surg. Today* 2000; 30:211-218.

[6] Hashmonai M, Shein M. Upper thoracic sympathectomy – open approaches. In: Paterson-Brown S, Garden J, Eds. Principles and Practice of Surgical Laparoscopy. WB Saunders, London. 1994; 587-603.

[7] Bernard C. Sur les effets de la section de la portion céphalique du grand sympathique. *Comptes. Rend. Soc. Biol.* 4:168-70, 1852.

[8] Alexander W. The treatment of epilepsy. Y J Pentland, Edinburgh. 1898; p.27-106.

[9] Jaboulay M. Le traitement de quelques troubles trophiques du pied et de la jambe par la dénudation de l'artère fémorale et la distension des nerfs vasculaires. *Lyon Med*. 1899; 91:467-468.

[10] Kotzareff A. Résection partielle du tronc sympathique cervical droit pour hyperhidrose unilatérale (regions faciale, cervicale, thoracique et brachiale droites). *Rev. Med. Suisse. Rom*. 1920; 40:111-113.

[11] Adson AW, Brown GE. Raynaud's disease of the upper extremities; successful treatment by resection of the sympathetic cervicothoracic and second thoracic ganglions and the intervening trunk. *JAMA* 1929; 92:444-449.

[12] White JC, Smithwick RH, Allen AW, Mixter WJ. A new muscle splitting incision for resection of the upper thoracic sympathetic ganglia. *Surg. Gynecol. Obstet.* 1933; 56:651-657.

[13] Smithwick RH. Modified dorsal sympathectomy for vascular spasm (Raynaud's disease) of the upper extremity. A preliminary report. *Ann. Surg.* 1936; 104:339-350.

[14] Lemmens HAJ. Thoracic resympathectomy. *Int Angiol* 1982; 1:147-148.

[15] Goetz RH, Marr JAS. The importance of the second thoracic ganglion for the sympathetic supply of the upper extremities – two new approaches for its removal. *Clin. Proc.* 1944; 3:102-114.

[16] Palumbo LT. Anterior transthoracic approach for upper thoracic sympathectomy. *Arch. Surg.* 1956; 72:659-666.

[17] Atkins HJH. Sympathectomy by the axillary approach. *Lancet* 1954; 1:538-539.

[18] Atkins HJB. Peraxillary approach to the stellate and upper thoracic sympathetic ganglia (letter). *Lancet* 1949; 2(254):1152.

[19] Telford ED. The technique of sympathectomy. *Br. J. Surg.* 1935; 23:448-450.

[20] Hughes J. Endothoracic sympathectomy. *Proc. Roy. Soc. Med.* 1942; 35:585-586.

[21] Kux E. 1239 cases of thorascopic sympathectomy and vagotomy; preliminary report. *Dtsch. Med. Wochenschr* 1953; 78:1590-1592.

[22] Kux M. Thoracic endoscopic sympathectomy in palmar and axillary hyperhidrosis. *Arch. Surgery* 1978; 113:264-266

[23] Spolianski G, Hashmonai M, Rudin M, Abaya N, Kaplan U, Kopelman D. Video-assisted open supraclavicular sympathectomy following air embolism. *JSLS* 2012; 16:337-339.

[24] Tögel B, Greve B, Raulin C. Current therapeutic strategies for hyperhidrosis: a review. *Eur. J. Dermatol.* 2002; 12:219-223.

[25] Atkins JL, Butler PEM. Hyperhidrosis: a review of the current management. *Plast. Reconstr. Surg.* 2002; 110:222-228.

[26] Eisenach JH, Atkinson JLD, Fealay RD. Hyperhidrosis: evolving therapies for a well-established phenomenon. *Mayo. Clin. Proc.* 2005; 80:657-666.

[27] Walling HW, Swick BL. Treatment options for hyperhidrosis. *Am. J. Clin. Dermatol.* 2011; 12:285-295.

[28] Schneider P, Moraru E, Kittler H, Binder M, Kranz G, Voller B, Auff E. Treatment of focal hyperhidrosis with botulinum toxin type A: long-term follow-up in 61 patients. *Br. J. Dermatol.* 2001; 145:289-293.

[29] Wilkinson HA. Percutaneous radiofrequency upper thoracic sympathectomy. *Neurosurgery* 1996; 38:715-725.

[30] Adler O, Englel A, Sargeno D. Palmar hyperhidrosis treated by percutaneous transthoracic chemical sympathicolysis. *Eur. Radiol.* 1994; 4:57-62.

[31] Hashmonai M, Assalia A, Kopelman D. Thoracoscopic sympathectomy for palmar hyperhidrosis: ablate or resect? *Surg. Today* 2001; 15:435-441.

[32] Woollard HH, Norrish RE. The anatomy of the peripheral sympathetic nervous system. *Br. J. Surg.* 1933; 21:83-103.

[33] Ehrlich E Jr, Alexander WF. Surgical implications of upper thoracic independent sympathetic pathways. *Arch. Surg.* 1951; 62:609-614.

[34] Kuntz A, Alexander WF, Furcolo CF. Complete sympathetic denervation of the upper extremity. *Ann. Surg.* 1938; 107:25-31.

[35] Hyndman OR, Wolkin J. Sympathectomy of the upper extremity. Evidence that only the second dorsal ganglion need be removed for complete sympathectomy. *Arch. Surg.* 1942; 45:145-155.

[36] Ray BS, Hinsey JC, Geohegan WA. Observations on the distribution of the sympathetic nerves to the pupil and upper extremity as determined by stimulation of the anterior roots in man. *Ann. Surg.* 1943; 118:647-655.

[37] Smithwick RH. The rationale and technic of sympathectomy for the relief of vascular spasm of the extremities. *N. Engl. J. Med.* 1940; 222:699-703.

[38] Atlas LN. The role of the second thoracic spinal segment in the preganglionic sympathetic innervation of the human hand – surgical implications. *Ann. Surg.* 1941; 114:456-461.

[39] Greenhalgh RM, RosEnglarten DS, Martin P. Role of sympathectomy for hyperhidrosis. *Br. Med. J.* 1971; 1:332-334.

[40] Lemmens HAJ. Importance of the second thoracic segment for the sympathetic denervation of the hand. *Vasc. Surg.* 1982; 16:23-26.

[41] O'Riordain DS, Maher M, Waldron DJ, O'Donovan B, Brady MP. Limiting the anatomic extend of upper palmar sympathectomy for primary palmar hyperhidrosis. *Surg. Gynecol. Obstet.* 1993; 176:151-154.

[42] Wong CW. The second thoracic sympathetic ganglion determines palm skin temperature in patients with essential palmar hyperhidrosis. *J. Auton. Nerv. Syst.* 1997; 67:121-124.

[43] Haxton HA. Treatment of hyperhidrosis. *Br. Med. J.* 1948; 1:636-639.

[44] Jochimsen PR, Hartfall WG. Peraxillary upper extremity sympathectomy: technique reviewed and clinical experience. *Surgery* 1972; 71:686-693.

[45] Keaveney TV, Fitzgerald PAM, Donnelly C, Shanik GD. Surgical management of hyperhidrosis. *Br. J. Surg*. 1977; 64:570-571.

[46] Shich CJ, Wand YC. Thoracic sympathectomy for hyperhidrosis. Report of 457 cases. *Surg. Neurol.* 1978; 10:291-296.

[47] Ellis H. Transaxillary sympathectomy in the treatment of hyperhidrosis of the upper limb. *Am. Surg*. 1979; 45:546-551.

[48] Welch E, Geary J. Current status of thoracic sympathectomy. *J. Vasc. Surg*. 1984; 1:202-214.

[49] Conlon KC, Keaveny TV. Upper dorsal sympathectomy for palmar hyperhidrosis. *Br. J. Surg*. 1987; 74:651.

[50] Golucke PJ, Garrett WV, Thompson JE, Talkington CM, Smith BI. Dorsal sympathectomy for hyperhidrosis – the posterior paravertebral approach. *Surgery* 1988; 103:568-572.

[51] Hashmonai M, Kopelman D, Kein O, Schein M. Upper thoracic sympathectomy for primary palmar hyperhidrosis: long-term follow-up. *Br. J. Surg*. 1992; 79:268-271.

[52] Yoon DH, Ha Y, Park YG, Chang JW. Thoracoscopic limited T-3 sympathicotomy for primary hyperhidrosis: prevention for compensatory hyperhidrosis. *J. Neurosurg*. (Spine 1) 2003; 99:39-42.

[53] Licht PB, Pilegaard HK. Severity of compensatory sweating after thoracoscopic sympathectomy. *Ann. Thorac. Surg*. 2004; 78:427-431.

[54] Deng B, Tan QY, Jiang YG, Zhao YP, Zhou JH, Ma Z, Wang RW. Optimization of sympathectomy to treat palmar hyperhidrosis: the systematic review and meta-analysis of studies published during the past decade. *Surg. Endosc*. 2011; 25:1893-1901.

[55] Lai YT, Yang LH, Chio CC, Chen HH. Complications in patients with palmar hyperhidrosis treated with transthoracic endoscopic sympathectomy. *Neurosurgery* 1997; 41:110-113.

[56] Kopelman D, Hashmonai M. The correlation between the method of sympathetic ablation for palmar hyperhidrosis and the occurrence of compensatory hyperhidrosis: a review. *World J. Surg*. 2008; 32:2343-2356.

[57] Baumgarten FJ, Reyes M, Sarisyan GG, Iglesias A,Reyes E. Thoracoscopic sympathicotomy for disabling palmar hyperhidrosis: a prospective randomized comparison between two levels. *Ann. Thor. Surg*. 2011; 92:2015-2019.

[58] Balsalobre RM, Mata NM, Izquierdo RR, Valverde FJA, Lòpez-Rodo LM, de Andrés JJR, Fernández JLG, Carretero MAC, Loscertales MC, Carbajo MC. Guidelines on surgery of the thoracic sympathetic nervous system. *Arch. Bronchoneumol.* 2011; 47:94-102.

[59] Cerfolio RJ, de Campos JRM, Bryant AS, Connery CP, Miller DL, DeCamp MM, McKenna RJ, Krasna MJ. The Society of Thoracic Surgeons' expert consensus for the surgical treatment of hyperhidrosis. *Ann. Thorac. Surg.* 2011; 91:1642-1648.

[60] Kopelman D, Hashmonai M, Schick C. The surgical treatment of hyperhidrosis. *Ann. Thorac. Surg.* 2012; 93:1019-1020

[61] Satyapal KS, Singh B, Partar P, Ramsaroop L, Pather N. Thoracoscopy: a new era for surgical anatomy. *Clin. Anat.* 2003; 16:538-541.

[62] Chung IH, Oh CS, Koh KS, Kim HJ, Paik HC, Lee DY. Anatomic variations of the T2 nerve root (including the nerve of Kuntz) and their implications for sympathectomy. *J. Thorac. Cardiovasc. Surg.* 2002; 123:498-501.

[63] Wong CW. Transthoracic video endoscopic electrocautery of sympathetic ganglia for hyperhidrosis: special reference to localization of the first and second ribs. *Surg. Neurol.* 1997; 47:224-230.

[64] Kopelman D, Hashmonai M. The appropriate level of sympathetic ablation for primary palmar hyperhidrosis. *Ann. Surg.* 2008; 248:687.

[65] Zhu LH, Wand W, Yand S, Chen L, Li D, Zhang Z, Chen S, Cheng X, Chen L, Chen W. Transumbilical thoracic sympathectomy with an ultrathin flexible endoscope in a series of 38 patients. *Surg. Endosc.* 2013; 27:2149-2155.

[66] Rua JFM, Jatene FB, de Campos JRM, Monteiro R, Tedde ML, Samano MN, Bernardo WM, Das-Neves-Pereira JC. Robotic versus human camera holding in video-assisted thoracic sympathectomy: a single blind randomized trial of efficacy and safety. *Interact. Cardiovasc. Thorac. Surg.* 2009; 8:195-199.

[67] Turner BG, Gee DW, Cizginer S, Konux Y, Karaca C, Willingham F, Mino-Kenudson M, Morse C, Rattner DW, Brugge WR. Feasibility of endoscopic transesophageal thoracic sympathectomy. *Gastrointest. Endosc.* 201; 71:171-175.

[68] Lin CC, Telaranta T. Lin-Telaranta classification: the importance of different procedures for different indications in sympathetic surgery. *Ann. Chirurg. Gynecol.* 2001; 90:161-166.

[69] Malone PS, Duigan JP, Hederman WP. Transthoracic electrocoagulation (T.T.E.C.) – a new and simple approach to upper limb sympathectomy. *Irish Med. J.* 1982; 75:20-21.

[70] Göthberg G, Claes G, Drott C. Electrocautery of the upper thoracic sympathetic chain: a simplified technique. *Br. J. Surg.*1993; 80:862.

[71] Hederman WP. Endoscopic sympathectomy. *Br. J. Surg.* 1993; 80:687-688.

[72] Elia S, Guggino G, Mineo D, Vanni G, Gatti A, Mineo TC. Awake one stage thoracoscopic sympathectomy for palmar hyperhidrosis: a safe outpatient procedure. *Eur. J. Cardiothorac. Surg.* 2005; 28:312-317.

[73] Drott C, Göthberg G, Claes G. Endoscopic procedures of the upper-thoracic sympathetic chain. *Arch. Surg.* 1993; 128:237-241.

[74] Haimovici H, Hodes R. Preganglionic nerve regeneration in completely sympathicomized cats. *Am. J. Physiol.* 1940; 128:463-466.

[75] Murray JG, Thompson JW. Collateral sprouting in response to injury of the autonomic nervous system and its consequences. *Br. Med. Bull* 1957; 13:213-219.

[76] Bengel FM, Ueberfuhr P, Schiepel N, Nexolla SG, Reichart B, Schwaiger M. Effect of sympathetic reinnervation on cardiac performance after heart transplantation. *N. Engl. J. Med.* 2001; 345:731-738.

[77] Orteu CH, McGregor JM, Almeyda JR, Rustin MHA. Recurrence of hyperhidrosis after endoscopic transthoracic sympathectomy – case report and review of the literature. *Clin. Exper. Dermatol.* 1995; 20:230-233.

[78] Hsu CP, Chen CY, Hsia JY, Shai SE. Resympathectomy for palmar and axillary hyperhidrosis. *Br. J. Surg.* 1998; 85:1504-1505.

[79] Kao MC. Transthoracic endoscopic sympathectomy. *Surg. Endosc.* 2001; 15:222.

[80] Lin TS. Video-assisted thoracoscopic "resympathectomy" for palmar hyperhidrosis: analysis of 42 cases. *Ann. Thor. Surg.* 2001; 72:895-898.

[81] Kopelman D, Hashmonai M, Ehrenreich M, Bahous H, Assalia A. Upper dorsal thoracoscopic sympathectomy for palmar hyperhidrosis: improved intermediate-term results. *J. Vasc. Surg.* 1996; 24:194-199.

[82] Freeman RK, van Woerkom JM, Vyverberg A, Ascioti AJ. Preoperative endoscopic sympathectomy for persistent or recurrent palmar hyperhidrosis. *Ann. Thorac. Surg.* 2009; 88:412-417.

[83] Licht PB, Clausen A, Landegaard L. Resympathicotomy. *Ann. Thorac. Surg.* 2010; 89:1087-1090.

[84] Ross JP. Sympathectomy as an experiment in human physiology. *Br. J. Sur.* 1933; 21:5-19.

[85] Shelley WB, Florence R. Compensatory hyperhidrosis after sympathectomy. *N. Engl. J. Med.* 1960; 263:1056-1058.

[86] Shoenfeld Y, Shapiro Y, Machtiger A, Magazanik A. Sweat studies in hyperhidrosis palmaris and plantaris. A survey of 60 patients before and after cervical sympathectomy. *Dermatologica* 1976; 152:257-262.

[87] Plaes EG, Függer R, Herbst F, Fritsch A. Complications of endoscopic thoracic sympathectomy. *Surgery* 1995; 118:493-495.

[88] Gjerris F, Olesen HP. Palmar hyperhidrosis. Long-term results following high thoracic sympathectomy. *Acta. Neurol. Scand.* 1975; 51:165-172.

[89] Cloward RB. Hyperhidrosis. *J. Neurosurg.* 1969; 30:545-551.

[90] Kim WO, Kil HK, Yoon KB, Noh KU. Botulinum toxin: a treatment for compensatory hyperhidrosis of the trunk. *Dermatol. Surg.* 2009; 35:833-838.

[91] Kopelman D, Assalia A, Ehrenreich M, Ben-Amnon Y, Bahous H, Hashmonai M. The effect of upper dorsal thoracoscopic sympathectomy on the total amount of body perspiration. *Surg. Today* 2000; 30:1089-1092.

[92] Denny-Brown D, Brenner C. Lesion of peripheral nerve resulting from compression by spring clip. *Arch. Neurol. Psychiat.* 1944; 52:1-19.

[93] Harold KL, Pollinger H, Matthews BD, Kercher KW, Sing RE, Heniford BT. Comparison of ultrasound energy, bipolar thermal energy, and vascular clips for hemostasis of small-, medium-, and large-sized arteries. *Surg. Endosc.* 2003; 17:1228-1230.

[94] Yanagihara TK, Ibrahimiye A, Harris C, Hirsch J, Gorenstein LA. Analysis of clamping versus cutting of T3 sympathetic nerve for severe palmar hyperhidrosis. *J. Thorac. Cardiovasc. Surg.* 2010; 140:984-989.

[95] Lin CC, Mo LR, Lee LS, Ng SM, Hwang MH. Thoracoscopic block by clipping – a better and reversible operation for treatment of hyperhidrosis palmaris: experience with 326 cases. *Eur. J. Surg.* 1998; 580:13-16.

[96] Reisfeld R. Sympathectomy for hyperhidrosis: should we place the clamps at T2-T3 or T3-T4? *Clin. Auton. Res.* 2006; 16:384-389.

[97] Kwang CW, Choi SY, Moon SW, Cho DG, Kwon JB, Sim SB, Wang YP, Jo KH. Short-term and intermediate-term results after unclipping: what happened to primary hyperhidrosis and trunkal reflex sweating after unclipping in patients who underwent endoscopic thoracic

sympathetic clamping? *Surg. Laparosc. Endosc. Percutan. Tech*. 2008; 18:469-473.

[98] Loscertales J, Congregado M, Jimenes-Merchan R, Gallardo G, Trivino A, Moreno S, Loscertales B, Galera-Ruis H. Sympathetic chain clipping for hyperhidrosis is not a reversible procedure. *Surg. Endosc*. 2012; 26:1258-1263.

[99] Candas F, Gorur R, Haholu A, Yiyit N, Yildizhan A, Gezer S, Sen H, Isitmangil T. The effect of clipping on thoracic sympathetic nerve in rabbits: early and late histopathological findings. *Thorac. Cardiovasc. Surg*. 2012; 60:280-284.

[100] Telaranta T. Secondary sympathetic chain reconstruction after endoscopic thoracic sympathicotomy. *Eur. J. Surg*. 1998; Suppl 580:17-18.

[101] Latif MJ, Afthinos JN, Connery CP, Perin N, Bhora FY, Chwajol M, Todd GJ, Belsley SJ. Robotic intercostal nerve graft for reversal of thoracic sympathectomy: a large animal feasibility model. *Int. J. Med. Robotic*. 2008; 4:258-262.

[102] Haam SJ, Park SY, Paik HC, Lee DY. Sympathetic nerve reconstruction for compensatory hyperhidrosis after sympathetic surgery for primary hyperhidrosis. *J. Korean. Med. Sci*. 2010; 25:597-601.

[103] Wong RHL, Ng CSH, Wong JKW, Tsang S. Needlescopic video-assisted thoracic surgery for reversal of thoracic sympathectomy. *Interact. Cardiovasc. Thorac. Surg*. 2012; 14:350-352.

[104] Scheib J, Höke A. Advances in peripheral nerve regeneration. *Nat. Rev. Neurol*. 2013; 9:668-676.

[105] Krarup C, Archibald SJ, Madison RD. Factors that influence peripheral nerve regeneration: an electrophysiological study of the monkey median nerve. *Ann. Neurol*. 2002; 51:69-81.

[106] Archbald SJ, Shefner K, Krarup C, Madison RD. Monkey median nerve repaired by nerve graft or collagen nerve guide tube. *J. Neurocsci*. 1995; 15:4109-4123.

[107] Kim DT, Luthringer DJ, Lai AC, Suh G, Czer L, Chen LS, Chen PS, Fishbein MC. Sympathetic nerve sprouting after orthotopic heart transplantation. *J. Heart Lung. Transplant*. 2004; 23:1349-1358.

[108] Kiyochi H, Ono A, Yamamoto N, Ohnishi K, Shimahara Y, Kobayashi N. Extrinsic sympathetic reinnervation after intestinal transplantation in rats. *Transplantation* 1995; 59:328-333.

[109] Meagher S, McGeachie J, Prendergast F. Vein to artery grafts. An experimental study of reinnervation of the graft wall. *Ann. Surg.* 1984; 200:153-158.

[110] Cowen T, Thrasivoulou C, Shaw SA, Abdel-Rahman TA. Transplanted sweat glands from mature and aged donors determine cholinergic phenotype and altered density of host sympathetic nerves. *J. Auton. Nerv. Syst.* 1996; 60:215-224.

[111] Hansen JM, Abildgaard U, Fogh-Andersen N, Kanstrup IL, Bratholm P, Plum I, Strandgaard S. The transplanted human kidney does not achieve functional reinnervation. *Clin. Sci.* (London) 1994; 87:13-20.

[112] Hyochi N, Kihara K, Arai G, Kobayashi T, Sato K. Reconstruction of the sympathetic pathway projecting to the prostate by nerve grafting in the dog. *BJU Int.* 2004; 94:147-152.

[113] Purves D, Thompson W, Yip JW. Re-innervation of ganglia transplanted to the neck from different levels of the guinea-pig sympathetic chain. *J. Physiol.* 1981; 313:49-63.

[114] Kocyigit P, Akay BN, Saral S, Akbostanci C, Bostanci S. Unilateral hyperhidrosis with accompanying contralateral anhidrosis. *Clin. Dermatol.* 2009; 34:e544-e546.

[115] Kopelman D, Hashmonai M, Assalia A, Bahous H. Primary palmar hyperhidrosis presenting with unilateral symptoms: a report of two cases and review of the literature. *Cardiovasc. Surg.* 1998; 6:94-96.

[116] Valley MA, Rogers JN, Gale DW. Relief of recurrent upper extremity sympathetically-maintained pain with contralateral sympathetic blocks: evidence for crossover sympathetic innervation? *J. Pain.* 1995; 10:396-400.

[117] de Campos JRM, Kauffman P, de Campos Werebe E, Filho LOA, Kusniek S, Wolosker N, Jatene FB. Quality of life, before and after thoracic sympathectomy: report on 378 operated patients. *Ann. Thor. Surg.* 2003; 76;886-891.

[118] Amir M, Arish A, Weinstein Y, Pfeffer M, Levy Y. Impairment in quality of life among patients seeking surgery for hyperhidrosis (excessive sweating): preliminary results. *Isr. J. Psychiatry Relat. Sci.* 2000; 37:25-31.

[119] Kumagai K, Kawase H, Kawanishi M. Health-related quality of life after thoracoscopic sympathectomy for palmar hyperhidrosis. *Ann. Thorac. Surg.* 2005; 80:461-466.

[120] Cinà CS, Robertson SGW, Young EJM, Cartier B, Clase CM. Effect of endoscopic sympathectomy for hyperhidrosis on quality of life using the illness intrusiveness rating scale. *Minerva Chir*. 2006; 61:231-239.

[121] Panhofer P, Zacherl J, Jakesz R, Bischof G, Neumayer C. Improved quality of life after sympathetic block for upper limb hyperhidrosis. *Br. J. Surg*. 2006; 93:582-586.

[122] Koskinen LOD, Blomstedt P, Sjöberg RL. Predicting improvement after surgery for palmar hyperhidrosis.

[123] Wolosker N, Yazbek G, de Campos JRM, Munia MA, Kauffman P, Jatene FB, Peuch-Leao P. Quality of life before surgery is a predictive factor for satisfaction among patients undergoing sympathectomy to treat hyperhidrosis. *J. Vasc. Surg*. 2010; 51:1190-1194.

[124] Stefaniak TJ, Proczko M. Gravimetry in sweating assessment in primary hyperhidrosis and healthy individuals. *Clin. Auton. Res*. 2013; 23:197-200.

[125] Elkeeb R, Hui X, Chan H, Tian L, Maibach HI. Correlation of transepidermal water loss with skin barrier properties in vitro: comparison of three evaporimeters. *Skin. Res. Technol*. 2010; 16:9-15.

[126] Edelberg R. Relation of electrical properties of skin to structure and physiologic state. *J. Invest. Dermatol*. 1977; 69:324-327.

[127] Ellaway PH, Kuppuswamy A, Nicotra A, Mathias CJ. Sweat production and the sympathetic skin response: improving the clinical assessment of autonomic function. *Auton. Neurosci*. 2010; 155:109-114.

[128] Lang E, Foerester A, Pfannmüller D, Handwerker HO. Quantitave assessment of sudomotor activity by capacitance hygrometry. *Clin. Auton. Res*. 1993; 3:107-115.

[129] Krogstadt AL, Piechnik SK. Are patients better than laboratory in assessing sweating? Validation study. *Dermatol. Surg*. 2005; 31:1434-1439.

[130] Henteleff HJ, Kalavrouziotis D. Evidence-based review of the surgical management of hyperhidrosis. *Thorac. Surg. Clin*. 2008; 18:209-216.

Index

B

C

D

E

F

G

H

I

J

K

L

Q

R

S

T

U

V

W

Y